The Political Economy of the Hospital in History

Edited by Martin Gorsky, Margarita Vilar-Rodríguez
and Jerònia Pons-Pons

Published by University of Huddersfield Press

University of Huddersfield Press
The University of Huddersfield
Queensgate
Huddersfield HD1 3DH
Email enquiries university.press@hud.ac.uk

First published 2020
Text © 2020 their respective authors

This work is licensed under a Creative Commons Attribution 4.0 International License

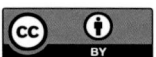

Images © as attributed

Every effort has been made to locate copyright holders of materials included and to obtain permission for their publication.

The publisher is not responsible for the continued existence and accuracy of websites referenced in the text.

All rights reserved. No part of this book may be reproduced in any form or by any means without prior permission from the publisher.

A CIP catalogue record for this book is available from the British Library.
Print: ISBN 978-1-86218-186-1

COVER IMAGE:
Clinic of Gynaecology, University of Szeged, 1931
© RF 750A/FA003/160/3058 Courtesy of the Rockefeller Archive Center

Acknowledgements

The editors gratefully acknowledge financial support from the European Union, the European Regional Development Fund (ERDF), and Spain's Ministry of Science and Innovation -State Research Agency- for the project entitled 'The historical keys of hospital development in Spain and its international comparison during the twentieth century', ref. RTI2018-094676-B-I00. The editors also thank the University of Huddersfield and the Wellcome Trust (under Medical Humanities Investigator Award grant no. 106720/Z/15/Z) for their financial support. We are also particularly grateful to Barry Doyle for arranging publication with Huddersfield University Press and to Robert Piggott for preparing the manuscript.

Contributors

Barry Doyle (University of Huddersfield)
Martin Gorsky (London School of Hygiene and Tropical Medicine)
Frank Grombir (University of Huddersfield)
Melissa Hibbard (University of Huddersfield)
Beatrix Hoffman (Northern Illinois University)
Axel C. Hüntelmann (Charité – University Medicine Berlin)
Anne Mills (London School of Hygiene & Tropical Medicine)
Ana Nemi (Federal University of São Paulo/Unifesp School of Philosophy, Languages and Human Sciences)
Jerònia Pons-Pons (University of Seville)
Balazs Szelinger (University of Huddersfield)
Margarita Vilar-Rodríguez (University of A Coruña)
Jin Xu (Peking University)

Contents

iii	Acknowledgements
vii	List of Figures and Tables
1	Introduction *Martin Gorsky, Margarita Vilar-Rodríguez and Jerònia Pons-Pons*
17	1. The historical creation of the hospital system in Spain: private hospital sector strategies in relation to the development of the public system *Margarita Vilar-Rodríguez and Jerònia Pons-Pons*
61	2. Charity and Philanthropy in the History of Brazilian Hospitals *Ana Nemi*
95	3. Principles and Problems of Hospital Funding in Germany in the Twentieth Century *Axel C. Hüntelmann*
137	4. The development of hospital systems in new nations: Central Europe between the Two World Wars *Barry Doyle, Frank Grombir, Melissa Hibbard and Balazs Szelinger*

181   5. Public, private and voluntary hospitals:
       economic theory and historical experience
       in Britain, c.1800-2010
       Martin Gorsky

221   6. The American Hospital: Charity, Public Service,
       or Profit Centre?
       Beatrix Hoffman

251   7. The rise of hospital centrism in China,
       1835-2018, from the perspective of financing
       Jin Xu and Anne Mills

294   Biographical Notes on Contributors

List of Figures

Figure 1.1 Interior view of "blood hospital" during the Spanish Civil War — 30

Figure 1.2 Illustrated scale model of the Residencia Francisco Franco (Barcelona) — 38

Figure 4.1 Relative Proportion of Provision in Hospitals and Mental Institutions 1931 — 148

Figure 4.2 Hospitals in Hungary, 1938 — 152

Figure 4.3 Plan for new Hospital and Medical School, Prague, 1937 — 159

Figure 4.4 Plans for Berehovo Provincial Hospital, Ruthenia, 1933 — 169

Figure 5.1 A conceptual model of hospital sectors in time — 184

Figure 7.1 Composition of sources of total health expenditures in China from 1978 to 2016 — 270

Figure 7.2 Pharmaceutical expenditures on outpatient and inpatient care — 273

Figure 7.3 Health expenditures by types of facility (adjusted to 1990 price level) — 277

Figure 7.4a Number hospitals classified by size (number of beds) (2002 and 2016) — 278

Figure 7.4b Estimated proportion of beds in hospitals classified by size (number of beds) (2002 and 2016) — 279

List of Tables

Table 1.1 General charity hospitals existing on 30 March 1886 — 22

Table 1.2 Charitable Establishments financed with private funds — 24

Table 1.3 'Residencias Sanitarias 'of the National Welfare Institute (INP) — 33

Table 1.4 Transformations of the public and private hospital map in Spain — 36

Table 1.5 Hospitals and beds in Spain according to property ownership — 45

Table 1.6 Public and private hospital facilities in 1977 — 47

Table 2.1 Assets and Liabilities of Sao Paolo Hospital 1960-1984 — 79

Table 4.1 Ethnic Population of Czechoslovakia, Poland and Hungary, percentage distribution, 1921-31 — 143

Table 4.2 Number of Hospitals and Beds in Czechoslovakia, Hungary and Poland, 1918-37 — 149

Table 4.3 Hospital beds by type, Czechoslovakia 1921 — 154

Table 4.4 Hospitals in Poland by Provider, 1927 and 1937 — 156

Table 5.1 Numbers and Percentage Distribution of Hospital Beds by Type (excluding asylums) 1861-1938 — 189

Table 5.2 Private Medicine under the NHS, UK 1955-2009 — 198

Table 5.3 NHS hospital beds and inpatients, 1951—2009/10 — 200

Table 5.4 Current health expenditure (public and private) as share (%) of gross domestic product, UK and comparator nations — 206

Table 7.1 Financial sources of hospitals and primary care providers (1928-1949) — 262

Table 7.2 Policy statements on ownership of and financial responsibility for primary care facilities — 269

Introduction[1]

Martin Gorsky, Margarita Vilar-Rodríguez
and Jerònia Pons-Pons

Hospitals are at once the site of the clinical encounter, the locus of medical teaching and research, and a cornerstone of health insurance and the welfare state. For medical historians, then, the study of the hospital must be multi-faceted, and in this book our perspective is that of political economy. Our starting point is the transformation undergone by health services during the twentieth century into one of the fastest growing economic sectors. While the level of health expenditures in rich countries was probably about 1% of GDP in 1900, it had risen (according to OECD statistics) to 4-6% in 1970 and to 10% or more by 2015.[2] Emerging economies have recently followed the trend, with, for example, health expenditures between 1995 and 2014 rising from 4% to 6% of GDP in China and 4% to 5% in India.

Much of these rising costs were consumed by the hospital service, with all its demanding requirements. Some were material and institutional, with heavily capitalised infrastructure, cutting-edge technologies, and highly trained professionals. Some were social and symbolic, in the costs of delivering health security and meeting political promises of access and provision. Hence the hospital's historical importance lay partly in its capacity to promote different economic activities and employment, not just medical care, but also the construction industry and the myriad administrative and ancillary services. And it lay partly in the policy arena, in which the relationship of competition and cooperation between public and private constituted an ongoing focus of political debate.

Despite their importance, and notwithstanding many single-institution histories, there are few historical studies that analyse the growth of hospital systems in major countries, their characteristics and their role within larger health care and welfare states. Lack of sources, complexity, and heterogeneity in their creation may partly explain this relative scarcity. The focus so far has been largely on Europe, with the German[3] and French cases[4] especially noteworthy, while the peculiarities of the British voluntary hospital have been much explored.[5] Outside Europe there are classic studies from the United States[6] and more recent contributions on the hospital system in Japan[7], China[8] and Sub-Saharan Africa.[9]

Such studies have laid the groundwork for conceptualising emergent hospital systems in ways that transcend national stories. Different forms took precedence depending on time and place, but broadly a mixed economy of health care was initially prevalent, with some combination of charity, state action and private payment. In Western Europe, the Anglosphere and Latin America, there seems to have been a mix of philanthropy and tax funding for public hospitals, and increasingly various types of mutual sickness insurance concerned with income replacement and primary care. Some countries had more comprehensive social health insurance of the type pioneered in Germany from 1883, including hospital cover. In colonial settings, the mixed economy could combine missionary medicine, private facilities for industrial workers, and state hospitals that addressed the needs, or fears, of European populations. For non-Western countries with indigenous medical practices, the growth of the public hospital was also shaped by the encounter with biomedicine, and the decisions taken about how this episteme should be incorporated with existing traditions.

By the mid-twentieth century, these diverse hospital trajectories were transformed into more integrated and regulated systems. Different factors combined to bring this about: the unprecedented levels of wealth now available to finance social costs in the advanced economies; the universalist political doctrines of socialism and liberal democracy; the imperative of 'development' that infused West/South relations in the late-colonial and early Independence era; and the broad authority attributed to biomedicine and its technologies over other modes of healing. In the rich countries there was a transition either to tax-based national health services, first piloted in New Zealand from 1938, or to one of two basic models of health insurance, the state social insurance arrangements mostly prevailing in Western Europe, or the private/non-profit approaches that took precedence in the United States.[10] Henceforth, European hospital systems would be heavily determined by the prevailing modes of coverage, the balance of insurance or tax-funding, and the mix of public and private ownership.[11] Meanwhile, in the United States, with private insurance much more prominent and commercial interest groups highly influential, the hospital system grew progressively more costly, while remaining less inclusive.[12]

In some poorer nations, development funding began to build hospital provision and to establish local training capacity, though in many places the legacy of colonial geographies meant institutional concentration in urban centres.[13] Yet while the high-income countries now drove towards universalism and planned hospital systems, in much of the world expansion was elusive. The economic take-off on which self-sustaining social expenditure was premised proved hard to achieve, as relationships of underdevelopment reasserted themselves. Improvement to hospital systems therefore took second place to infectious disease programmes or improving access to selective aspects of primary care.[14]

By the end of the twentieth century access to hospitals in most European Union countries was through a universal compulsory health insurance scheme within a broader social protection system. However, private health insurance had become increasingly important, either complementing or supplementing state packages.[15] The context was one of neo-liberal philosophies, waves of privatisations, retrenchment and the ongoing fiscal crisis of welfare states: all have been bitterly contested in the arena of health politics. Thus, while the foothold of private insurance in the hospital market is common across OECD countries, this varied (2002) from 92% population coverage in the Netherlands (where it was highly regulated), to 13% in Spain and 10% in the UK. In the United States the eventual expansion of health cover under social security, through Medicare and Medicaid for older and poorer populations, had not resolved inequities of hospital access, and recurrent reform efforts were politically inflammatory.[16] In China, the unleashing of private enterprise after Mao's death saw increasing commercialisation of the hospital, and earlier social protection systems undermined, especially for rural populations.[17] The dominance of the World Bank over development policies in low-income countries anxious for debt relief imposed the 'Washington consensus': that purely statist welfare models were dysfunctional and that plural forms hospital provision, financed more extensively from user fees were the way forward.[18] For such places the century closed with fierce debate on whether this 'structural adjustment' had brought negative effects, and with the grail of universal health coverage still far off.

In sum, then, the work of medical and welfare historians has provided a broad chronological and conceptual framework within which to write the history of hospital systems. The aim of this book is to interrogate this framework further, through a series of studies that range over time and space. Specifically, we are interested in the variations between places in the structure and organisation of hospital systems, the balance between public and private sectors, and the politics attending this. These problems break down into subsidiary objectives, which the authors tackle. From a public and private perspective, why and how were medicine, health and hospitals transformed? To what extent were the different national trajectories of the twentieth century determined by earlier configurations of funding and ownership? Why did a hospital model based on private institutions gain ascendency in some countries while state-built hospitals took precedence in others? What was the historical relationship between public and private hospitals over time: did they collaborate or compete? To what extent was the development of hospital systems conditioned by economic and political factors?

Analysis of the financing and administration of different hospital systems raises a conceptual challenge. How exactly should hospital scholars seeking a shared language for comparative discussion delineate 'public' and 'private'? Our cases show that 'public' hospitals could have non-statutory income sources, and that 'private' hospitals ranged from commercial to non-profit, with many different shades between. Here we begin with a definition of public hospitals as being the property of the central, regional or local state. We also distinguish between private hospitals created as profit-making companies and those constituted as charitable institutions financed by private foundations. The chapters will bring into view the national variants and consider how far they acted in a complementary or a competitive fashion.

With respect to timeframe, our initial suggestion that authors began their accounts in the late-1800s proved both helpful and misleading. Clearly the hospital underwent 'medicalisation' at some point, transforming it from an institution with limited therapeutic efficacy that sheltered the terminally ill, sustained the poor, and gave spiritual aid, into something else. For some, the later nineteenth century seems the moment that the modern hospital emerged, albeit retaining the tradition of refuge offering bed rest and nursing, but now also a diagnostic centre exploiting observational and laboratory techniques, locus of new therapies, grounded in biomedical sciences, and all staffed by medical professionals and qualified auxiliaries.[19] Others though have found in histories of case selection, of record keeping, and of the language and gaze of the physician, evidence of much earlier beginnings.[20] Alongside these narratives of Western modernity, as we will see, run others from across the globe, which observed their own chronologies. For example, the interplay between a biomedical profession in the making, a hospital sector combining healing, proselytising and social control, and the needs of the state, could shape such factors as the balance of primary or institutional care, or the persistence of charitable status across several centuries.

Today's health care debates and the present economic uncertainties make this a salient moment to consider from a historical perspective the hospital networks constructed by different states. To date we do not have a historical analysis that provides an overall explanation of their geographical development, their capacity of coverage, their singularities in international terms and their main deficiencies. Thus, in general terms, all the chapters include the following aspects: a first part establishing the historical hospital inheritance at least from the late nineteenth and early twentieth centuries, and in some cases significantly earlier; followed by explanation of the different stages of growth in the twentieth century, with emphasis on models, financing, construction and institutional aspects that conditioned pathways of hospital development, on its journey to become a necessary part of the twentieth-century welfare state.

Composition of the book

Our historical case studies begin with Spain and Brazil, to observe hospital models rooted in early modern charitable practices, where politics and pace of economic development forestalled moves to universalism until quite late in the twentieth century.

The Spanish case analysed by Vilar-Rodríguez and Pons-Pons initially bore similarities to other European countries, with limited systems inherited from *Ancien Régime* charity and then perpetuated by liberal governments. This comprised a public hospital sector that combined charity and limited state budgets, as well as institutions linked to municipal and provincial councils, and a private realm of hospitals and asylums run as charitable foundations. Obsolete in terms of fabric and equipment, this only began to change from the 1920s with the emergence of hospitals founded by industrial businesses, friendly societies and insurance companies, as well as clinics and polyclinics created by entrepreneurial doctors for the middle class. Spain's Civil War (1936-9) and subsequent Franco dictatorship (1939-75), meant its path diverged somewhat from Northern Europe, where integrated social security systems meant a move towards universal coverage. While the fascists introduced compulsory sickness insurance (1942) and a Health Care Facilities Plan, which led to the creation of an expensive new system, these moves were not responses to demand or redistributive equity. Instead they served propaganda purposes and compensated the groups and regions that had supported the regime. Meanwhile insufficiency of public beds favoured the private system, which collaborated in the management of the state health insurance. By the late 1960s, pressure from urbanisation and population growth on the fragmented, understaffed and technologically backward hospital network was stalled by lack of funding and political paralysis: Spain did not even have a Ministry of Health until 1977. With the transition to democracy health care coverage became a right under the 1978 Constitution, and in 1986 the country's health care and hospital model was redefined after decades of underinvestment and uneven growth.

Nemi's study of Brazil, a Portuguese colony until 1822, similarly reveals long-term processes shaping the configuration of its hospital system. Despite the creation of a national health service by legislation in 1988, these survivals make aspects of the Brazilian model more similar to the United States, with private hospitals claiming public funds, tax exemption privileges, and organisational autonomy. This trajectory, Nemi shows, dates to the colonial era when the *misericordia* organised health care through voluntary donations and enjoyed privileges granted by the Portuguese Crown. These structuring foundations substantially persisted after Brazilian independence in 1822, as the experience of the Hospital of the São Paulo Holy House of Mercy demonstrates. Such institutions, and similar philanthropic hospitals in the later nineteenth century, negotiated tax exemption rates for providing free health care to the poor, combining private charity with public resources from municipal councils. Behind this public/private interplay lay the interest of local elites – initially landowning but increasingly business and medical – to maintain a field of economic and social power that allowed them to shape urban development. Moving into the twentieth century, Nemi takes the teaching hospital of the São Paulo School of Medicine as emblematic. The enduring integration of public and private/philanthropic sectors persisted into the era of social insurance, and beyond to the 1988 Constitution which permitted such hospitals to enter service provision contracts with the public health service. Couched within neoliberal discourse about the inefficiency of the public sector these have remained a vehicle for the persistence of private medicine, the undermining of universalism, and the diversion of public funds and resources to support patients with private health insurance.

Next we move to Germany, where the archetypal form of social health insurance was pioneered, and to Central Europe, where the successor states created after the First World War saw hospital policy as an aspect of nation-building.

Hüntelmann begins by noting the chorus of concern in Germany since the 1960s about the deficiencies of hospital financing, which have inflicted a near-perpetual reign of cost-containment reforms.

Although such debates appear relatively new, they are, he contends, only the latest iteration of a discourse originating in the early nineteenth century when the hospital became 'modern'. After tracing these beginnings, he sets out the impact of Germany's statutory health insurance system from the 1880s, then describes how hospital finance changed over the twentieth century. The interrelationship between health insurance and hospital funding has wrought significant changes in the character of the hospital. Most fundamental were the transition from a charitable to a medical and public institution at the end of the nineteenth century, and that from welfare institution to public enterprise in the last decades of the twentieth. This has shifted the role of the hospital, he argues, from an institution primarily responsible to the community, into a profit-orientated enterprise, in which health has too often been reduced to a cost-factor in debates about ailing public finances.

A narrower chronology is taken by Doyle, Grombir, Hibbard & Szelinger, who explore the creation of hospital systems in interwar Central Europe. Their interest is the new nations which emerged following the collapse amidst revolution and defeat in 1918 of the three multinational empires that had hitherto dominated this region. Concentrating on Poland, Czechoslovakia and a much-truncated Hungary, they show how they sought to utilise health care, and especially hospital provision, as evidence of their progressivism and modernity, and as a symbol of nationhood. Yet their intentions were constrained by a complex health inheritance, persistent financial crises and significant health challenges, especially in their poverty-stricken eastern regions. Blending research in national archives with international perspectives from the League of Nations and the Rockefeller Foundation, they examine the provision and extent of institutional care, how its institutions and patients were financed, and how the multi-ethnic character of these nations impacted on hospital policy and its role in nation building. While each country put considerable effort, resource and political will into creating national health care systems, financial weakness, ethnic conflict and urban rural divisions limited their choices and curtailed expansion and modernization. This analysis, Doyle, Grombir, Hibbard & Szelinger argue, contrasts revealingly with the rather teleological 'road to the welfare state' narratives which mark Western hospital histories of this same period.

Studies of the Anglophone countries, Britain and the United States then follow, their systems apparently not dissimilar at the end of the nineteenth century, but subsequently diverging dramatically.

The well-researched British case has long been a historiographical reference for the hospital in a system that culminated in the post-war welfare state. Gorsky utilises this familiar framework in a new way, to interrogate the proposition from welfare economics that the market, the state and the voluntary sector each have demonstrable virtues and limitations as providers of social goods. Can the dynamics of 'market failure', 'state failure' and 'voluntary failure' explain changing preferences for modes of hospital provision through time? Taking a long-run view, he addresses four key questions. First how do we explain the pattern of growth of the hospital up to the mid-twentieth century, with its distribution between private, public and voluntary sectors? The private hospital sector seems always to have been small, and through the nineteenth century the state emerged as the dominant provider thanks to its default role in managing populations that fell outside the labour market; the smaller voluntary sector meanwhile circumvented the stigmatising aspects of state provision for the respectable poor, while also serving a social function for donors. Second he examines the major system reform c.1942-48, when the National Health Service brought hospitals under the central state. Voluntary failures and the inequities of local government partly account for this, but explanation also includes the displacement effect of war, the role of the labour movement, the capacity of the British state, and path dependent processes. Third he accounts for the late twentieth century decline of the hospital, and its changing distribution between public and private sectors. State failure does not adequately explain these changes: deinstitutionalisation of psychiatric care was also driven by changing therapeutic management, while the rise of the private hospital followed deliberate and contingent political decisions. Finally, he appraises the emergence of an active policy of management of the state hospital sector from the 1960s, arguing that evidence for failure lay not with the intrinsic nature of public administration, but with the periodic tendency towards underfunding.

The different path taken across the Atlantic is revealed in Hoffman's discussion of the United States, whose hospital system trajectory was unlike other Western nations. While it has both public and private hospitals, the latter are supported with extensive public subsidies while maintaining an ideology of private control and rejection of 'government interference'. The consequent implications for access to care, public accountability, and patient voice have created what Rosemary Stevens called the 'essential historical dilemma' of American hospital politics. Hoffmann examines this interleaving of public and private, first sketching the blurred distinction between public and private sectors after government subsidies rescued private hospitals during the Great Depression. A massive increase in federal funding of private hospital construction following World War Two, and the establishment of the Medicare and Medicaid programmes in 1965, further increased the scale of taxpayer subsidies to the private hospitals, whose insistence on autonomy from government control was mostly accepted by Congress. This process, Hoffmann shows, created serious obstacles to access, for example through the funding for segregated hospitals in the U.S. South that allocated services based on race. It also contributed to inefficiency, inequity and massive cost inflation, notably through the Medicare programme, which until the 1980s allowed private hospitals to set their own fees. Yet she also finds examples of citizens utilizing federal programmes to demand greater access to care: the medical civil rights movement's protest at segregated hospitals in the 1960s; Medicaid recipients' law suits against hospitals that refused to accept poor patients in the 1970s; and the establishment of a right to emergency care in 1986. The chapter concludes with the impact of the 2010 Affordable Care Act ('Obamacare') which provides federal subsidies to the private health insurance industry and expands Medicaid coverage for low-income people, bringing hospitals millions of newly insured patients. It thus embodies the same public-private paradox.

The book closes with China, whose case demonstrates the adoption of the biomedical hospital in a great power undergoing rapid modernisation, in conditions of intense political upheaval. Xu and Mills begin by pointing out that although China was once considered an international model for low-cost rural primary health care, this reputation was founded on a short-lived combination of factors. Over the long term, China has instead suffered from chronic concentration of high-quality resources in its hospitals, despite recurrent efforts to strengthen primary care. Their chapter analyses the historical evolution of both hospitals and primary care in China from the perspective of financing, in a study covering the period 1835-2018. It shows that the developmental trajectories for earlier models of hospital and primary care diverged between 1835 and 1949, with low-cost primary care emerging only after the establishment of relatively elitist hospitals. The divergence was consolidated, they argue, between 1949 and 1978, giving rise to two different models with contrasting fiscal space, service-finance methods and administrative policies. After 1978, market-based financing mechanisms brought direct competition for patients and resources between hospitals and primary care providers, and exposed the weakness of the latter. Pharmaceuticals and technologies became critical vehicles for hospitals' revenue generation. Increasingly, available resources were absorbed primarily by hospitals, while primary care continued to be under-resourced. Overall, the study sheds light on how historical health financing influences in China have shaped contemporary challenges in finding the appropriate balance of care to serve the population.

Together, the chapters enable us to advance the historical world map of the construction of the different hospital models. While our authors do not make specific use of path dependence theory, they do emphasise the impact of diverse institutional frameworks in defining national health systems, and the long-term reach of these influences. Their comparative perspective advances understanding of the complexities involved in each country, and each branch of the hospital system and brings new evidence to the current debate on health care models, financing and health reforms. This book, with the encouragement it gives to comparative and cooperative research, aims to allow us to find better answers to that deceptively simple, and engrossingly complex question: what is the hospital?

1. Margarita Vilar-Rodríguez and Jerònia Pons gratefully acknowledge financial support from the European Union, the European Regional Development Fund (ERDF), and Spain's Ministry of Science, Innovation and Universities for the project entitled "The historical keys of hospital development in Spain and its international comparison during the twentieth century", ref. RTI2018-094676-B-I00

2. Pierre-Yves Donzé and Paloma Fernández, 'Health Industries in the Twentieth Century. Introduction', *Business History, Special Issue*, 61, 3 (2019), 385-403.

3. Sussane Hilger, 'Welfare Policy in German Big Business after the First World War: Vereinigte Stahlwerke AG, 1926-33', *Business History*, 40, I (1998), 50-76. Axel C. Hüntelmann, 'The Birth of the Patient as a cost- and benefit-factor. Funding and Management of Hospitals in Germany in the 20th century', I International Workshop, The Construction, funding and management of the public and private hospital systems of developed countries (Seville, November, 2017).

4. Jean-Paul Domin, *Une histoire économique de l'hôpital (XIXe-XXe siècles). Une analyse rétrospective du développement hospitalier, Tome I (1803-1945)* (Paris: Comité d'histoire de la Sécurité Sociale, 2008); Christian Chevandier, *L'hôpital dans la France du XXe siècle* (Paris: Perrin, 2009)

5. Steven Cherry, 'Before the National Health Service: Financing the Voluntary Hospitals, 1900-1939', *The Economic History Review*, 50 (1997), 305-26; Martin Gorsky, John Mohan and Martin Powell, 'The Financial Health of Voluntary Hospitals in Interwar Britain', *Economic History Review*, 55 (2002), 533-57; Barry Doyle, *The Politics of Hospital Provision in Early Twentieth-Century Britain* (London: Pickering and Chatto, 2014).

6. Charles Rosenberg, *The Care of Strangers. The Rise of America's Hospital System* (New York: Johns Hopkins University Press, 1987). Rosemary Stevens, *In Sickness and in Wealth. American Hospitals in the Twentieth Century* (New York: Johns Hopkins University Press, 1989).

7. Pierre-Yves Donzé, 'Architects and knowledge transfer in hospital systems: The introduction of Western hospital designs in Japan (1918–1970)', *Business History, Special Issue*, 61, 3 (2019), 538-57.

8. Michelle Renshaw, 'The Evolution of the Hospital in Twentieth-Century China', in Bridie Andrews and Mary Brown Bullock (eds), *Medical Transitions in Twentieth-Century China* (Bloomington: Indiana University Press, 2014), 317-35.

9. Barbara McPake, 'Hospital Policy in Sub-Saharan Africa and Post-Colonial Development Impasse', *Social History of Medicine*, 22, 2 (2009), 341–60.

10. Bernard Harris and Paul Bridgen (eds), *Charity and Mutual Aid in Europe and North America since 1800* (New York: Routledge, 2007); Marcel Van der Linden (ed), *Social Security Mutualism: The comparative History of Mutual Benefit Societies* (Bern: Peter Lang, 1996); Martin Gorsky, 'The Growth and Distribution of English Friendly Societies in the Early Nineteenth Century', *The Econom-*

ic History Review, 51, 3 (1998), 489-511; David T. Beito, *From Mutual Aid to the Welfare State. Fraternal Societies and Social Services, 1890-1967* (Chapel Hill: The University of North Carolina Press, 2000); Brian J. Glenn, 'Understanding mutual Benefit societies, 1860-1960', *Journal of Health Politics, Policy and Law*, 26 (2001), 638-51; Bernard Harris, *The Origins of the British Welfare State: Social Welfare in England and Wales, 1800-1945* (Hampshire: Palgrave Macmillan, 2004); John E. Murray, *Origins of American Health Insurance. A History of Industrial Sickness Funds* (New Haven-London: Yale University Press, 2007); Michel Dreyfus, *Les assurances socials en Europe* (Rennes: Presses Universitaires de Rennes, 2009).

11. Melissa A. Thomasson, 'From Sickness to Health: The Twentieth-Century Development of the Demand for Health Insurance', *The Journal of Economic History*, 60, 2 (2000), 504-08. Harris and Bridgen, *op. cit.* (note 9); John Henderson, Peregrine Horden and Alessandro Pastore, 'Introduction. The World of the Hospital: Comparisons and Continuities', in John Henderson, Peregrine Horden and Alessandro Pastore (eds), *The impact of Hospitals 300-2000* (Bern: Peter Lang, 2007), 15-57; Dreyfus, *op. cit.* (note 10).

12. Murray, *op. cit.* (note 9); Thomasson, *op. cit.* (note 10); Christy F. Chapin, 'The American Medical Association, Health Insurance Association of America, and Creation of the Corporate Health Care System', *Studies in American Political Development*, 24, October (2010), 143–67; Christy F. Chapin, *Ensuring America's Health: The Public Creation of the Corporate Health Care System* (New York: Cambridge University Press, 2015).

13. Vicente Navarro, *Medicine Under Capitalism* (London: Croom Helm, 1976).

14. Randall M. Packard, *A History of Global Health: Interventions into the Lives of Other People* (Baltimore: Johns Hopkins University Press, 2016).

15. Elias Mossialos, Anna Dixon, Josep Figueras and Joe Kutzin (eds), *Funding health care: options for Europe* (Buckingham: Open University Press, 2002).

16. Paul Starr, *Remedy and Reaction: The Peculiar American Struggle Over Health Care Reform* (New Haven: Yale University Press, 2011).

17. Jane Duckett, *The Chinese State's Retreat from Health: Policy and the Politics of Retrenchment* (London: Routledge, 2011).

18. David de Ferranti, 'Paying for Health Services in Developing Countries: An Overview', *World Bank Staff Working Papers* (Washington, D.C.: World Bank, 1985).

19. Ole P. Grell, Andrew Cunningham and Robert Jütte (eds), *Healthcare and Poor Relief in 18th and 19th Century Northern Europe* (Aldershot: Ashgate, 2002). Henderson, Horden and Pastore (eds), *op. cit.* (note 11).

20. Michel Foucault, *The Birth of the Clinic: an archaeology of medical perception* (New York: Vintage, 1975). Laurence Brockliss and Colin Jones, *The Medical World of Early Modern France*, Oxford: Clarendon Press, 2004, 677, 689-700; Caroline Hannaway and Anne La Berge, *Paris Medicine: Perspectives past and present* (Amsterdam: Rodopi, 1998).

Chapter 1

The Historical Creation of the Hospital System in Spain: Private Hospital Sector Strategies in Relation to the Development of the Public System.[1]

Margarita Vilar-Rodríguez*
(University of A Coruña)

Jerònia Pons-Pons
(University of Seville)

Introduction

The available historiography has shown how the so-called mixed economy of welfare (co-existence of forms of solidarity, state action and private companies) was a preliminary step towards the creation of two basic models of health insurance in the mid-twentieth century: state insurance schemes prevailed in Western Europe, while private insurance companies predominated in the United States.[2] Thus, from a historical point of view, public health care systems that progressed towards universal coverage were prevalent in Western Europe, which prompted the construction of a solid network of publicly owned hospital infrastructure.

In particular, some studies have analysed the historical creation of public hospital systems in certain countries in Western Europe, driven by the passage of compulsory social insurance legislation and increasing state participation, and coinciding with a parallel decline in philanthropy and charity in the Western world.[3] Significant differences between countries are to be found within this general model, both in ways of funding and managing the system and in the historical configuration of the hospital map, depending on whether or not hospitals of different origin and specialisations were incorporated into the public network. On the other hand, there is the US model, where health and hospital care have historically been covered by private insurance companies. This has been explained in terms of a complex set of factors, especially the lobbying power of the private interest groups involved in this process in combination with other political interests and the preferences of professional doctors. Other factors include the increase in family income, the development of medical technology and government policies that consolidated private sector predominance through measures such as tax incentives.[4] In this respect, R. Stevens concludes that as a result of this historical evolution, the US hospital system has become unique: a combination of public and private institutions that are at once charities and businesses, social welfare institutions and icons of the country's science, wealth, and technical achievements.[5] Despite the cuts in public health systems in recent years, it seems to be beyond all doubt that the US model is a more expensive system in the long run, and less successful in meeting the needs of the chronically ill and the socially disadvantaged.[6]

Overall, the available literature on the creation of hospital systems in an international context provides us with three key lessons.[7] First, the danger of over-simplifying when classifying countries into the two large typical models related to Western Europe and the United States. It seems clear that the global scene is in fact much more complex, and even within Western Europe each country must essentially be considered as a unique case. Second, the importance of the public and private approach to analysing the historical development of hospital systems and the important implications in terms of efficiency, coverage and equity. Third, the relevance of the historical perspective, as different forms of hospital coverage had priority in each country according to the period and the adopted model. Here, factors such as expeditiousness in implementing state insurance schemes, social spending performance and the more recent initiation of privatisation processes within public health systems in some countries have led to changes to the original models and have produced a different historical fit, or correlation, between public and private hospital coverage, depending on the period analysed.

The case of Spain provides an excellent example for substantiating these three points. This country was one of the last in Western Europe to pass its first state sickness insurance (1942); it belatedly consolidated a universal public health system with the law of 1986; and it is an interesting case study of how a private hospital sector was capable of developing strategies in each historical stage to maintain (and expand) its market niche during the development of the public system. From the last third of the nineteenth century and throughout the twentieth century, the modern Spanish hospital system was fashioned over the course of different historical stages that may be examined by focusing on the interaction (whether collaborative or competitive) between public and private sectors. In this respect, the private hospital sector increased the private provision of hospital beds as a reaction to different factors. One was the emerging demand of the middle and working classes who were not covered by the country's public health institutions (including those run by municipal councils and provincial authorities known as *diputaciones*).[8] Others were the obligations imposed on employers due to the approval of regulations or social insurance schemes, and increasing medicalisation together with new medical or pharmacological techniques that were not provided by the public health system. Consequently, and for other reasons that are analysed in this chapter, during some periods the private hospital sector substituted for the public sector, in others complemented it, and at times both sectors were in competition with one another. As a result, a complex relationship between both sectors evolved that vacillated between necessary cooperation and logical competition.

With respect to the hospital classification criterion, due to historical tradition and the (not very abundant) sources available, the Spanish historiography has been based on whether hospitals were publicly or privately owned in order to analyse the long-term development of the hospital system.[9] This article follows this tradition, categorising hospitals as being under public or private ownership. In this case, hospitals built and financed by public institutions are included in the public sector. On the other hand, privately owned hospitals include those of the Church, the Spanish Red Cross (*Cruz Roja*), private charitable institutions—similar to the British voluntary hospitals—and private profit-seeking hospitals. This classification according to type of ownership remained essentially unchanged until 1986. Although property ownership is quite clear, the type of funding and the groups of patients admitted by each type of hospital are much less obvious. In particular, it is difficult to distinguish between the charitable foundations of privately-owned hospitals, which in theory covered poor patients, and the private profit-orientated hospitals which were based on business and market criteria and treated paying patients. This difficulty is rooted in the fact that, over time, the private charity hospitals increased the number of beds dedicated to paying patients, while a similar process also occurred with the hospitals belonging to the Church and the Red Cross. Meanwhile, some private profit-seeking hospitals dedicated a few working hours a week to treating poor patients, on the grounds of Christian charity. Owing to these blurred distinctions, we feel that property ownership is a much clearer guideline for the Spanish case.

The creation of the hospital system before the passage of state insurance (1880-1936)

Between 1880 and 1936, the public/charitable hospital network in Spain remained antiquated and tied to the limited state, provincial, and municipal budgets and only treated the population classified as poor. These institutions had limited therapeutic efficacy and their main aim was to provide shelter for the sick poor, most of them chronically or terminally ill, who did not have the support of a family care network.[10] It must be borne in mind that the welfare system of the *Ancien Régime* in Spain, based on religious charity, was transformed in the nineteenth century by means of the disentailment laws, which liquidated a large part of Church property and transferred the management of many of its hospital establishments to state, provincial and municipal authorities (General Charity Law of 20 June 1849).[11] However, provincial and local charity had sparse resources during this period. Thus, their main efforts were concentrated on providing food, clothing and hospital attention for the poorest families, and on the confinement of the old, vagrants and foundlings in hospices and children's homes.[12] On the other hand, general charity establishments under state management were few in number, funded by small items in the general state budget, alms and royal subsidies, and most of them were located in the capital, Madrid.

Table 1.1: General charity hospitals existing on 30 March 1886

Name	City	Purpose of the institution	No. of beds
Hospital de la Princesa	Madrid	For the sick of both sexes with acute non-infectious disorders*	200
Hospital de Jesús Nazareno	Madrid	To house disabled and incurable women	250
Hospital de Nuestra Señora del Carmen	Madrid	To house disabled and incurable men	250
Hospital del Rey	Toledo	To house the decrepit and blind of both sexes	120

Source: Statistical Yearbook of Spain (*Anuario Estadístico de España*), Reseña geográfica y estadística de España, 1888, 1030-1.
* Note: On one hand, an acute patient would be a patient at risk of death, who needed urgent treatment and, in some cases, an urgent surgical operation. On the other hand, a chronic patient would be a patient who needed lifelong treatment, in some cases with hospital admission.

Provincial authorities, however, were obliged by the Charity Law of 1822/36 (the first law regulating this area in Spain) to establish four charitable establishments in each province: a *Casa de Maternidad y Expósitos* (maternity and foundling home), a *Casa de Socorro* (emergency medical and surgical treatment), a *Casa de Misericordia* (home for children and the elderly) and a public hospital (in most cases treating infectious patients).[13] In fact, hospitals exercised a crucial police function for the maintenance of public order; that is to say, to remove children, vagrants and old people from the streets by means of confinement in hospices, asylums and refuges. Moreover, as noted above, provincial councils inherited some of the disentailed hospitals. In 1909, official figures registered 183 provincial charitable establishments operating throughout the country.[14] As for town and city councils, they managed an old network, part of it of medieval origin and the rest inherited from the disentailment of ecclesiastical property, comprising modest establishments of charitable aid.[15] Many of these establishments disappeared in the second half of the nineteenth century due to a lack of resources. Sources accounted for 363 charitable institutions run by municipal authorities to treat the sick in 1909.[16]

Altogether, the charitable establishments of the provincial and municipal councils provided a total of 66,014 beds in Spain in 1909, which was equivalent to a ratio of 3.3 beds per thousand inhabitants.[17] Most of these beds were used for asylum purposes and not for surgical treatment or medical care; in fact, a significant part of the funds of these institutions was used for providing food for the sick rather than for curing them. The population with an official certificate of poverty (which identified a person without minimal resources or the capacity to obtain them) had priority to be treated in these institutions free of charge.[18] In 1909, the census of poor families in Spain showed the figure of 813,815 (around 3.25 million inhabitants if we take into account an average of approximately four members per family). Meanwhile, there was a total of 7,769 doctors in charitable establishments in 1909, which was equivalent to a ratio of 418 poor people per practitioner.[19] However, they were unequally distributed geographically and thus, in rural areas and in the smaller municipalities, infectious or more seriously ill patients were sent to hospital in the provincial capital. The cost of a poor sick person's stay was covered by the municipality where he or she was registered, which at times led to non-payment or disputes between the provincial commission and municipal councils.[20]

There were also hospitals classified as private charity (which belonged to the Church because they had not been disentailed or were privately owned) existing alongside this precarious network of public charity. These hospitals received private funds from their founders (income, public debt, urban and rural real estate), and they were managed by their patrons as foundations (voluntary hospitals). Private charity had its own legislative framework.[21] According to official statistics, there were 337 private charitable hospitals in Spain in 1886, concentrated above all in three provinces: Barcelona (41), Navarre (36) and Cordoba (33).

Table 1.2: Charitable Establishments financed with private funds from their respective founders in 1886

Province	Hospital	Population*	Province	Hospital	Population*
Álava	-	102,494	León	4	354,737
Albacete	1	221,444	Lérida	-	330,677
Alicante	5	426,636	Logroño	19	184,073
Almería	-	352,946	Lugo	10	464,358
Ávila	8	176,769	Madrid	10	491,984
Badajoz	6	430,049	Málaga	4	490,826
Baleares	-	284,398	Murcia	13	427,208
Barcelona	41	749,443	Navarre	36	316,340
Burgos	21	387,856	Orense	-	394,638
Cáceres	3	303,700	Oviedo	-	588,031
Cádiz	3	417,346	Palencia	2	194,527
Canarias	-	267,036	Pontevedra	2	469,439
Castellón	5	288,921	Salamanca	6	281,511
Ciudad-Real	-	264,908	Santander	7	236,105
Córdoba	33	379,464	Segovia	16	134,262
Coruña	1	609,337	Seville	4	500,567
Cuenca	-	242,231	Soria	-	157,173
Gerona	-	322,631	Tarragona	-	341,601
Granada	2	478,347	Teruel	1	250,604
Guadalajara	9	211,249	Toledo	14	343,951

Province	Hospital	Population*	Province	Hospital	Population*
Guipúzcoa	11	176,297	Valencia	3	648,159
Huelva	-	191,303	Valladolid	15	255,438
Huesca	-	272,157	Vizcaya	-	183,098
Jaén	-	390,115	Zamora	21	262,524
			Zaragoza	1	403,362
Spain, Total	337	16,642,273			

Source: For hospitals see *Reseña geográfica y estadística de España*, 1888, 52, 1030-31. For population see Statistical Yearbook of Spain (*Anuario Estadístico de España*), 1866-1867, 53. *Inhabitants in December 1867.

The territorial distribution of these hospitals did not correspond to demographic criteria; the most populated provinces of the country did not have more establishments. Consequently, there were considerable territorial inequalities. We do not have data available on what kind of sick people were admitted, how many combined charitable care with paying patients, or how many focused exclusively on providing refuge for children, the elderly and the chronically and incurably sick. However, most of them were run by trusts comprised of members of the medical class and the urban patriciate.

The patrons defended the classification of their hospitals as private charity, and themselves as benefactors, in order to obtain more freedom in their management, but also to take advantage of tax exemptions and other benefits. One of the most paradigmatic cases is that of Hospital de Santa Creu in Barcelona, which was the city's only hospital for more than five hundred years and a benchmark scientific institution in the country. An order of 15 September 1853 declared it a public and provincial establishment. Nevertheless, in the following decades the managers who ran the hospital fought to convert it into a private charity hospital and thereby prevent Barcelona's financial authorities from carrying out an operation to confiscate its property and assets. On 18 June 1874, the Directorate General for Charity, Health and Penitentiary Establishments (*Dirección General de Beneficencia, Sanidad y Establecimientos Penitenciarios*) revoked the public classification and declared Hospital de Santa Creu a private charity establishment.[22] This reclassification enabled the hospital's patrons to regularly apply for exemption from paying the taxes levied on the assets of legal persons, which contributed to the preservation of its considerable assets, beyond the control of the public authorities.[23] These assets were further increased by means of bequests and raffles.[24] Over time, these institutions, without losing the charitable category that benefited them fiscally, increased their supply of pay beds and, in future stages, especially from 1942, participated in economic agreements with public institutions to cover the demand for beds in the public hospital system.

This public and private hospital network proved to be increasingly insufficient in the light of Spain's economic, urban and industrial development from the late nineteenth century, within a framework of growing social demands, notable among which were calls for the extension and improvement of health coverage for the population as a whole.[25] This process was accompanied by advances in bacteriological research, especially from the 1870s onwards, which opened the way to significant progress in the care and treatment of transmissible diseases (tuberculosis, cholera, diphtheria and malaria). This in turn led to the need to create new facilities such as laboratories and diagnostic devices. Within this context, the function of hospitals changed, and Spain was no exception. Some of the old hospitals, now obsolete, were demolished (*Hospital de San Juan de Dios* in 1897), others were renovated (*Hospital Provincial de Madrid*) and, in some cases, transferred to new locations (*Hospital del Buen Suceso* was founded in 1583 and transferred to a new site in 1885, and Hospital de los Franceses was created in 1615 and relocated in 1881). This process of change also included the creation of clinical hospitals with a heavy focus on teaching and research linked to universities and training. Thus, *Hospital Clínico de Madrid* (founded by the central state) became a university hospital in the first decades of the twentieth century and the clinical hospital in Barcelona, work on which had commenced in 1881, was opened in 1906. Meanwhile, as regards public hospitals, despite limited resources and within a system that was archaic in terms of both management and materials, a number of important research and teaching initiatives led by prominent specialists emerged in diverse surgical specialities. This was the case, for example, of the *Instituto de Terapéutica Operatoria*, founded in 1880 by the surgeon Federico Rubio y Galí as a department—with two wards of twenty beds for men and women—within the obsolete *Hospital de la Princesa* in Madrid.[26] This institute played a key role in the training of doctors and nurses during the 1880s in a context of high mortality, especially infant mortality, in Spain as a whole, but also in Madrid.[27]

However, in the first three decades of the twentieth century, the main problem relating to hospital coverage in Spain lay in the high percentage of the population that was not officially registered poor (*pobre de solemnidad*) but also could not afford to pay for health care services. This was the case of two large segments of the population: the growing mass of urban labourers along with the urban middle class, and the vast population engaged in agriculture (around half of the active population). The latter group had to make do with the archaic system of coverage provided by rural municipal hospitals or provincial hospitals. Consequently, workers who were not treated by these hospitals turned to friendly societies to seek medical attention, even though this usually entailed no more than primary medical care due to the limited resources of most of these institutions. There were exceptions, however, such as the dense network of Catalan friendly societies that was able to create a small hospital network. In 1939, the Federación de Mutualidades de Cataluña (Federation of

Mutual Benefit Societies in Catalonia) encompassed 1,023 affiliated mutual societies with a total of 334,881 members.[28] Some of these (*La Quinta de Salud La Alianza, Mutual Salus, Clínic Rabasa* and *Alianza Mataronense*, among others) provided clinic and hospital services without a time limit for patients' stays.[29]

Industrial employers, for their part, obliged by law to treat employees injured in accidents as from 1900, promoted small clinics providing trauma surgery and associated specialties by means of mutualism or insurance contracts. Large companies in sectors with significant accident rates—mining and the railways—acted more directly by establishing and financing their own hospital systems through foundations or local institutions. This was the case of the hospital in Riotinto, Huelva, and the Triano mining hospitals (Gallarta, Matamoros and El Cerco) in Biscay province.[30] Finally, doctors who worked in public or private charitable hospitals frequently funded small, specialised clinics to meet a growing demand for new varieties of surgical coverage from the middle classes and insurance companies and mutuals. The increase in small clinics was especially significant in Catalonia and the Basque Country—the most industrialised regions and with a greater percentage of urban population—founded by urologists, gynaecologists and other specialists. These clinics incorporated diagnostic advances such as laboratories and X-rays and further improvements including electric lighting in operating theatres, ventilation and aseptic wards. Clinics and polyclinics offered modernisation in comparison with the outdated public hospitals and attracted the middle and upper classes. Examples of this process include *Clínica San Ignacio* in Guipúzcoa (1906), and *Clínica Corachán* (1921), *Clínica Platón, Clínica San Jorge* and *Clínica Bretón* (1925) in Barcelona. In this way, private professional initiatives increased the supply of private beds as opposed to the public sector apathy during the period of Primo de Rivera´s Dictatorship (1923/30) rooted in charity and incapable of establishing a public health system similar to other Western European countries.[31] Political apathy, a lack of state resources due to an obsolete tax system, and opposition from the medical profession and private insurance companies delayed the introduction of a sickness insurance system that required new infrastructure and a substantial budget.[32] This led to better hospital coverage and more beds available in industrial regions, which in the long term created territorial inequalities in health care coverage.

The hospital system in Spain after the passage of compulsory public sickness insurance (1936/63)

The trend described above for the creation of the hospital map in Spain during the first decades of the twentieth century was interrupted by the Spanish Civil War (1936/9), which affected the medical class profoundly. An important element had to go into exile, thereby interrupting some clinical projects; others saw how their hospitals were destroyed or seriously damaged during the conflict that led to the establishment of the Franco Dictatorship (1939/75).[33] Under these circumstances, new political and propaganda propositions linked to National Catholicism (an ideology represented by the Falange, the single party of the fascist dictatorship) had a significant impact on the gestation process of the hospital system in Spain.[34] The Falangists maintained control of the Ministry of Labour (*Ministerio de Trabajo*), also responsible for social and family policies, and which entailed control of the National Welfare Institute (*Instituto Nacional de Previsión*; hereinafter INP), the managing body of the social insurance schemes. Using paternalistic language and intense propaganda, the Falange sought to win over the masses to its cause, proposing measures to protect the traditional Catholic family, through subsidies, birth rate and marriage prizes, and large-scale social projects, championed by the introduction of compulsory sickness insurance (*Seguro Obligatorio de Enfermedad*, hereinafter SOE). This form of insurance was one of the most desired by the population in the long, tough post-war period in Spain and it was the only social insurance that had not been legislated for before the Spanish Civil War, which added further value to the Falange's social project.

Figure 1.1: Interior view of one of the many buildings that were adapted as "blood hospitals" during the Spanish Civil War.

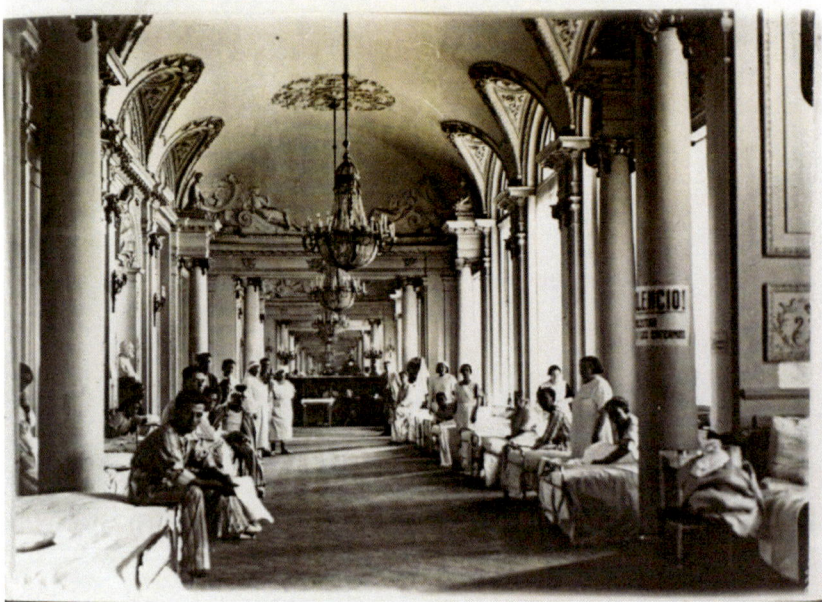

Source: Biblioteca Nacional de España, ref. GC-CAJA/114/14

The urgency of implementing this insurance scheme led to it being passed quickly in 1942. However, this was without an accompanying financial plan or sufficient infrastructure for its application.[35] Spain's precarious economic situation, characterised by autarky and the postwar economic crisis, obliged two important decisions to be taken. First, from the outset the insurance scheme was severely limited in terms of coverage of the population (it was initially only for the lowest-paid industrial workers in a country with a predominance of agricultural labourers)[36] and provisions (initially only general practitioners, with no specialities or hospital services apart from emergency surgery). In any case, insurance opened the door to a new form of health coverage for part of the population, unconnected with traditional charity (for the poor) and private health care (for those who could afford to pay for it). Second, in view of the lack of resources, senior figures at the Ministry of Labour decided to hand over management of the new health insurance to the private sector (including both private for-profit and non-profit mutuals) for over a decade. In return, the private sector provided the administration, medical staff and infrastructure (clinics and hospitals) required to cater for insured workers. In 1945, the collaborating bodies covered 55% of the companies affiliated to the SOE, comprising 77% of the insured. In 1955, coverage was still 40% and 64% respectively.[37] These management agreements were by no means free of tension between the private sector and Falange leaders who, from 1963, with an incipient but insufficient public hospital network, recovered public management of compulsory sickness insurance through the Basic Law of Social Security.

In order to achieve this control and consolidate its social project, in the 1950s the INP tried to implement its own National Healthcare Facilities Plan (*Plan Nacional de Instalaciones Sanitarias*). This plan envisaged the construction of a network of primary health care centres (outpatient clinics) and above all large hospitals (known as *'residencias sanitarias'*) throughout the country. Public hospitals surviving in the post-war period (state, provincial and municipal) were not used for the SOE or the Facilities Plan. This was a consequence of the power struggle between the INP—under the control of the Ministry of Labour, which was in the hands of Falange—and the Directorate General for Health (*Dirección General de Sanidad*, hereinafter DGS)—under the control of the Ministry of the Interior (*Ministerio de Gobernación*)—which was in the hands of the Catholic branch of the dictatorship's power groups. Many of these old hospitals continued, although with obsolete infrastructure, to provide charitable functions as refuges, under the control of the DGS, which was basically responsible for public hygiene and control of epidemics. This body was also charged with meeting the basic health care needs of rural Spain, beyond the scope of the INP's ambitious projects. In this way, the rural population was doubly marginalised by the dictatorship in terms of health care, as it was left on the side-lines with regard to both the coverage of the SOE and the construction of basic care facilities. This was especially significant if we bear in mind that Spain was predominantly an agrarian society in its production structure and distribution of employment until the 1960s.

The objectives of the Facilities Plan had to be reduced on several occasions due to the lack of material and financial resources in a country still hit by shortages and harsh living conditions. The large and spacious INP hospitals were built slowly, and many remained underused once the work was finished, due to a lack of human and material resources. Official sources show sixty-three *residencias sanitarias* built throughout Spanish territory with a capacity of almost 12,000 beds in a country with a population of 30.6 million; although probably in many cases the building work had still not been completed and others that were finished had not started functioning. Some reports from this time reveal that most of the hospitals built remained underused; some did not even have permanent staff or the organised provision of integrated services and specialities.[38] Furthermore, the administrative and executive management of health care facilities, including hospitals, under the umbrella of the INP was concentrated in a single body dependent on the Institute's provincial authority (*delegado provincial*). This arrangement gave preference to the political control of functions and relegated good resource management and the quality of services to second place. Moreover, the vast majority of directors or managers responsible for public health centres were 'health inspectors politically connected to the governing regime, or persons linked to the regime who always had the approval of the civil governor who was, at the same time, the Provincial Head of the Movement'.[39]

Table 1.3: 'Residencias Sanitarias'of the National Welfare Institute (INP) in 1963

Province	No.	Beds	Population	Beds per 1,000 inhab	Province	No.	Beds	Population	Beds per 1,000 inhab
Álava	1	144	138,934	1.04	Logroño	1	240	229,852	1.04
Albacete	1	190	370,976	0.51	Lugo	1	115	479,530	0.24
Alicante	1	363	711,942	0.51	Madrid	9	857	2,606,254	0.33
Almería	1	329	360,777	0.91	Málaga	1	307	775,167	0.40
Ávila	1	67	238,372	0.28	Murcia	0	0	800,463	0.00
Badajoz	1	424	834,370	0.51	Navarre	0	0	402,042	0.00
Baleares	2	398	443,327	0.90	Orense	1	23	451,474	0.05
Barcelona	2	773	2,877,966	0.27	Oviedo	3	688	989,344	0.70
Burgos	1	309	380,791	0.81	Palencia	1	100	231,977	0.43
Cáceres	1	217	544,407	0.40	Las Palmas	1	268	453,793	0.59
Cádiz	2	242	818,847	0.30	Pontevedra	1	250	680,229	0.37
Castellón	0	0	339,229	0.00	Salamanca	0	0	405,729	0.00
Ciudad-Real	2	46	583,948	0.08	Castellón	5	35	490,655	0.07
Córdoba	1	364	798,737	0.46	Santander	1	156	432,132	0.36
La Coruña	1	258	991,729	0.26	Segovia	0	0	195,602	0.00
Cuenca	0	0	315,433	0.00	Seville	1	593	1,234,435	0.48

Province	No.	Beds	Population	Beds per 1,000 inhab	Province	No.	Beds	Population	Beds per 1,000 inhab
Gerona	1	291	351,369	0.83	Soria	0	0	147,052	0.00
Granada	1	428	769,408	0.56	Tarragona	0	0	362,679	0.00
Guadalajara	1	148	183,545	0.81	Teruel	1	160	215,183	0.74
Guipúzcoa	1	330	478,337	0.69	Toledo	0	0	521,637	0.00
Huelva	1	304	399,934	0.76	Valencia	1	411	1,429,708	0.29
Huesca	0	0	233,543	0.00	Valladolid	1	310	363,106	0.85
Jaén	1	176	736,391	0.24	Vizcaya	1	600	754,383	0.80
León	2	53	584,594	0.09	Zamora	1	99	301,129	0.33
Lérida	1	254	333,765	0.76	Zaragoza	2	648	656,772	0.99
Spain Total	56	11.968	30,430,998	0.39					

Source: BOE, no. 140, 13 June 1966, 7389-427; Population from Statistical Yearbook of Spain (*Anuario Estadístico de España*), 1963, 455.

In general terms, the place and the programme to build each *Residencia Sanitaria* were decided according to political criteria based on the power and contacts of each provincial governor. These criteria resulted in territorial inequalities between population and beds (Table 1.3). All in all, bureaucratic management, scarce resources and precarious care provision converted each of these '*residencias sanitarias*' into a kind of large, underused polyclinic that performed its function inadequately. Basically, at the start of the 1960s, those affiliated to the SOE attended these hospitals for surgery, but for little else.[40] Consequently, the agreements with the private sector continued in force.

In any case, and in spite of the slow progress, the INP's '*residencias sanitarias*' gradually gained weight in Spain's hospital system and were treating a growing number of people, as the percentage of the population covered and the provisions offered by the SOE increased (Table 1.4). The number of public hospitals diminished compared with 1949 (1949: 737 and 1963: 589), but the number of beds increased (1949: 89,079 and

1963: 100,782). The drop in the number of hospitals was due, above all, to the closure of old hospitals of municipal and provincial charity. The increased number of beds was mainly due to the construction of large *'residencias sanitarias'* located in provincial capitals and other cities of high demographic concentration. Meanwhile, the state had also increased the number of hospitals for treating tuberculosis and other infectious diseases and mental hospitals under the direction of the DGS. The 'state' group also included hospitals attached to the Ministry of Education, which were, essentially, the clinical hospitals of the Faculties of Medicine, and prison health care institutions attached to the Ministry of Justice.[41] On top of these must be added the 48 military hospitals operating in Spain in 1963, created to treat troops and officers during times of peace and in wartime.[42] Finally, the number of hospitals under the control of the *Secretaría General del Movimiento* (SGM) of the Falange, which basically treated party members in the absence of other infrastructure, remained almost unchanged between 1943 (41) and 1963 (43).

With regard to the private hospital system from 1949 to 1963, the number of establishments increased between 1949 (885) and 1963 (1,037) along with the number of available beds, 38,264 and 52,109 respectively (Table 4). Altogether, the group of private hospitals accounted for almost sixty-six per cent of the total number existing in Spain in 1963. This group had a very diverse composition, and included clinics and hospitals founded by the Church (93), the Spanish Red Cross (*Cruz Roja*) (38), private benefactors (105), and two more that are difficult to categorise.[43] However, the most heterogeneous group of private hospitals in 1963 comprised those classified as 'privately owned' and which amounted to a total of 799 centres in this year. This increase was largely due to the converging interests of the government and the private sector. The development of maternity clinics was especially noteworthy within this group at a time when Spain initiated a historic 'baby boom' and the SOE did not have sufficient facilities to provide this service. Only one maternity hospital of the SOE appeared in the 1963 catalogue, managed by the INP and located in Madrid. Meanwhile, there were around thirty maternity centres under the control of municipal and provincial authorities (some of them successors to the old charitable maternity homes founded in the nineteenth century) and 107 private clinics specialised in maternity care. Meanwhile, the DGS, outside the Falange's control, catered to the needs of the rural population through the so-called *Centros Maternales de Urgencia* (emergency maternity centres), located in small municipalities or district centres. For any other type of medical care, the rural population had to travel to the nearest charitable provincial and/or municipal hospitals or otherwise pay for the services of a private clinic.

Table 1.4: Transformations of the public and private hospital map in Spain (in percentage)

	1949		1963		1981	
	1	2	1	2	1	2
Publicly Owned						
Military	9.09	20.48	8.15	14.05	9.05	7.90
State (P.N.A. y E.T., DGS, others)	17.37	20.43	27.84	25.79	1	2
INP	4.88	1.52	9.51	11.72	1	2
SGM	5.56	2.61	7.64	2.18	50.37	57.25
Provincial Council	19.00	41.56	20.37	39.37	26.41	31.39
Municipal Council	44.10	13.40	26.49	6.89	14.18	3.46
Total public (A). Number	737	89,079	589	102,250	409	130,298
Privately Owned						
Church	12.77	34.05	8.97	32.63	10.08	21.73
Spanish Red Cross	3.62	3.83	3.66	3.82	5.12	5.48
Private (profit-making and charitable)	83.62	62.12	87.37	63.55	84.81	72.79
Total private (B). Number	885	38,264	87.37	52,036	645	63,598

A in total (%)		45.44	69.95	36.22	66.28	38.80	67.20
B in total (%)		54.56	30.05	63.78	33.73	61.20	32.80
Total A+B. Number		1,622	127,343	1,626	154,268	1,054	193,896

Notes: 1. Number of establishments; 2. Number of beds. *It refers to inpatient units.
Source 1949: Statistical Yearbook of Spain (*Anuario Estadístico de España*), 1951, 684; Source 1963: *Boletín Oficial del Estado* (Official State Gazette) 13 June 1966, no. 140, 7389-427. In the 1963 catalogue hospital infrastructure in the colonies is also recorded: (Fernando Po (4), Río Muni (11) and Spanish Sahara (5); all under the presidency of the Government). This source also includes the hospitals of the *Secretaría General del Movimiento* (S.G.M.) and the *Patronato Nacional Antituberculoso y de las Enfermedades del Tórax* (P.N.A. y E.T.); Source 1981: Statistical Yearbook of Spain (*Anuario Estadístico de España)*, 1985, 709.

Overall, the hospital map in Spain from 1949 to 1963 shows three relevant trends. First, as regards publicly owned hospitals, there was a very significant fall in the number of old charitable hospitals managed by municipal and provincial institutions, an increase in the number of large hospitals and bed capacity of the INP (under the Facilities Plan) and a more modest growth in the number of hospitals under the DGS, specialising above all in treating infectious diseases such as tuberculosis, which had a great impact on Spain in the post-Civil War period. Finally, the number of military hospitals and the number of beds they provided fell around 30 per cent between 1949 and 1963. Second, with regard to privately owned hospitals, the Church reduced the number of hospitals it had operating (most dedicated to charitable functions and serving as refuges), while the number of private hospitals increased, driven by market opportunities and agreements signed with the SOE. Generally speaking, the hospitals providing shelter and charity lost weight in circumstances where some of their users were able to receive care or treatment under the SOE. Third, and paradoxically, the implementation of the sickness insurance scheme led to a fall in the number of public hospitals compared with private

Figure 1.2: Illustrated scale model of the Residencia Francisco Franco (Barcelona), the first "Residencia Sanitaria" (large hospital) inaugurated by the Franco dictatorship in 1955.

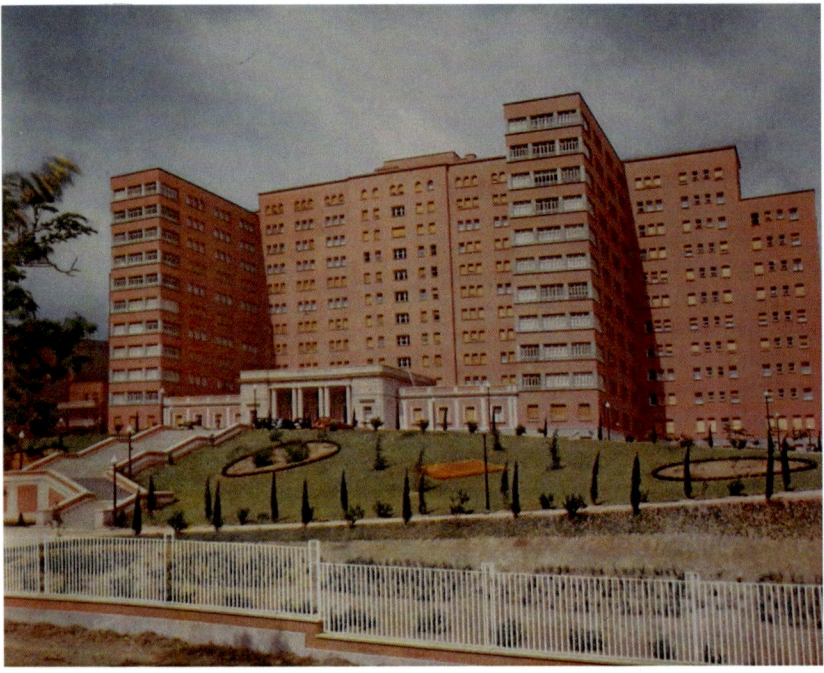

Source: Catálogo Plan de Instalaciones del Seguro Obligatorio de Enfermedad. Huarte y Cía, S.L. constructor.

hospitals, although there was a more comparable trend for both types in terms of the number of beds, due to the large capacity of the new hospitals built by the INP.

The 1960s saw some significant changes in the dictatorship's policies. The Falangists lost political power at the highest levels, and their capacity to mobilise the masses was diminished. The so-called technocrats took over most of the ministerial posts and the regime initiated the path laid down by the Stabilisation Plan of 1959, a plan dictated and financed to a large extent by the International Monetary Fund. In any event, health coverage was a goal to be achieved. Two decades after its introduction, there were now five million insured under the SOE, and around 7.5 million beneficiaries between direct insurance and the collaborating entities, which altogether accounted for thirty-nine per cent of the total population. During this initial period the limited public hospital network provided the private sector with a market niche, either by covering the population without any right to coverage, or through the signing of agreements by means of which the SOE was applied.

In summary, the system of social insurance introduced by the Franco dictatorship was an indispensable instrument within the overall strategy of propaganda and subjugation of the workers.[44] In particular, sickness insurance played a key role in the dictatorship for two fundamental reasons. First of all, before the Civil War, the state did not legislate, regulate or fund the area of health care provision, which remained in the hands of mutual societies and private companies. This resulted in substantial deficiencies in the coverage of the population. The dictatorship took advantage of the weakness of these institutions, and of the gap in state regulation of the risk of sickness, to convert this insurance into a key element of its political propaganda. Once the subordination of the workers had been achieved through the repressive measures that were imposed by means of strict labour regulation, it was necessary to ensure a certain degree of social stability. In order to achieve this aim, the regime needed to show a 'friendlier' face to workers. Social insurance and family policies, which included goals typical of fascist regimes such as encouraging a higher birth rate or defending maternity and the traditional family, fulfilled this role to perfection. The construction of hospitals fitted well into this framework.

Limited transformations of a hospital model in permanent imbalance in the last years of the dictatorship: 1963/75

The Spanish economy experienced strong growth in the 1960s, which was accompanied by a baby boom and a massive rural exodus. Population growth, urbanisation and improved living conditions brought new consumption habits and greater demand for health care, which highlighted the fragile public health and hospital system developed in previous decades. In particular, three major shortcomings came to light: a) health care philosophy was based on limited care in terms of coverage and provision, a model far removed from the universal health care existing in other European countries; b) funding, in view of the scarcity of public resources, encumbered by an archaic tax system inherited from the nineteenth century, and the prevalence of propaganda purposes in a dictatorship with insufficient political will to promote a modern hospital system; c) management, with underutilisation, lack of coordination and poor administration of available hospital establishments and services. In this regard, it is important to bear in mind the diversity of owners and management bodies of the public hospitals shared between the Ministry of Labour (to which the INP, managing body of the SOE, belonged), the Ministry of the Interior (to which the DGS belonged), the Ministry of Education (responsible for the clinical hospitals) and the Ministry of Justice and the Army (military hospitals). This complex map was completed by the provincial and municipal institutions that continued to manage most of the country's public charitable hospitals.

Within this context, two key laws for health coverage were passed: the law of 1962 regulating hospitals and the Basic Law of Social Security of 1963 (implemented in 1967). The former was intended to improve coordination between the various administrations and hospital networks existing at that time. However, a substantial part of this legislation was not implemented due to the lack of public health resources. Nevertheless, this paralysis did not block the process of building large public hospitals or a modest improvement in hospital care, above all in large cities. The law of 1963 was theoretically intended to pave the way towards universal health coverage, increase the state's financial contribution, and improve provision. In practice it consolidated a shared system, sustained by the social contributions of employers and workers (particularly onerous for the latter in a context of low wages), while at the same time it demonstrated that universalisation was not economically possible, for the time being.[45] Perhaps the main novelty of this legislation was the suppression of any possible profit-making intention of the managers of the social insurance schemes, which entailed the elimination of the agreements for the private management of the SOE. Consequently, health coverage progressed very slowly from 41.8% of the population in 1965 to 54.28% in 1970 and 61.74% in 1975, the last year of the dictatorship. This general system of coverage coexisted with other special regimes that provided health coverage to groups of workers excluded from the SOE (agriculture, marine workers, coal industry, services, self-employed etc.), either due to the resistance of employers, or the economic limitations of the insurance, or because they preferred to remain under a system that offered better coverage and provisions than the general regime (especially in the case of white-collar workers). On the other hand, 75.2% of public health expenditure was still funded through social contributions in 1980; financing through taxes only started to become predominant from 1989.[46] The problems of funding the public health system in general, and the hospital system in particular, made this insurance scheme one of the main destabilising elements of the Social Security accounts in Spain at this time.[47]

Despite all these difficulties, there were some significant developments in the hospital sector during this period. First, the INP tried to respond to the growing demand for coverage with the construction of *ciudades sanitarias* (large complexes comprising a group of adjacent independent buildings specialising in maternity, trauma and orthopaedics, children etc. that shared services such as laboratories, laundry or cafeteria).[48] Work on building *ciudades sanitarias* commenced in 1964 in the large provincial capitals: Madrid, Barcelona, Valencia, Seville, Zaragoza, Oviedo and Bilbao. In most cases (except Madrid and Valencia) these *ciudades sanitarias* were built around the large hospitals created under the Facilities Plan. This process reinforced the hospital-based health care model that was being established in Spain.[49]

Second, planning of hospitals in the new *ciudades sanitarias* was designed within a new organisational framework and with a renewed philosophy of health care as a public service, that is, as a right rather than as a work of charity. This was achieved thanks to the implementation of the Basic Law of Social Security of 1963.[50] In this situation, a paradigm shift occurred in the training of medical specialists. In the first decades of the twentieth century, most doctors trained as assistants of a skilled practitioner in the doctor's surgery or hospital.[51] In the 1950s, a new generation of doctors understood that in order to specialise with any degree of assurance it was necessary to go abroad, as they were not guaranteed adequate training in Spain. These doctors who travelled to the United States or countries in Western Europe became a key element in the modernisation of medicine in Spanish hospitals, both public and private, and in the introduction of new medical and surgical specialities. In particular, the training of doctors as specialists under the MIR medical internship system, based on 'learning by working', had originated at Johns Hopkins Hospital (Baltimore, USA) in the late nineteenth century and was incorporated into the Spanish hospital system in the 1960s by a group of doctors who had undertaken their specialist training in the United States.[52] Within this process, the percentage of doctors who worked in hospitals in Spain grew (1949: 32.8%, 1963: 39.7% and 1973: 68.4%).[53] The instigation of training programmes for medical specialists, the professionalisation of the body of nurses and assistant nurses as opposed to the voluntary and religious personnel present in a large number of hospitals, and the creation of a board of directors with a hospital manager of a more technical and professional nature, enabled the old *residencias sanitarias* to be transformed into more modern hospitals. Meanwhile, in order to train the management and administrative staff, the first training course for hospital managers was organised in 1967.[54] Third, and as part of this new strategy, the dictatorship promoted the inauguration of new university clinical hospitals geared towards teaching and training. Their objective was the renewal of education in the medical faculties and subsequent coordination with the Social Security.

The desire to modernise was present in all of these initiatives. However, progress was slow. In fact, what is seen is a Spanish hospital structure where two contradictory systems were forced to coexist.[55] First, there were still a considerable number of hospitals (above all of a charitable nature) operating under the old model from the previous stage, which were coexisting with new thriving (private and public) hospitals, with a heavy focus on teaching and research and a more professional management. That is to say, there was a problem of lack of integration, coordination, planning and the rational use of resources because there was no state institution that properly coordinated this complex hospital structure. Second, the new hospitals needed to expand their outpatient facilities while the old outpatient clinics needed hospitals. Third, there was an increase in the number of doctors trained through modern teaching programmes that did not find employment in the 'old' hospitals.[56] This enforced coexistence led to serious defects and aggravated the organisational crisis inherited from previous decades.

All in all, in the final years of the Franco dictatorship (1939-75), the Spanish hospital system was near to collapse, with three basic problems: insufficient coverage, provision and infrastructure;

heterogeneous strategic approaches and management; and funding problems.[57] These were three problems inherited from previous stages that were exacerbated in a situation where the hospital function had finally started to be modernised in Spain. The hospital map available for 1981 reveals the perpetuation of a model consisting of a constellation of numerous hospitals of different proprietorship and different stages of development. Nevertheless, the extension of coverage both in terms of provision and the number of insured, along with the increasing number of beds available in the *residencias sanitarias* of the SOE, weakened the role of the provincial, and especially the municipal, public charitable hospitals, which in 1981 showed a decline in number and in beds compared with the preceding period (Table 4). Nevertheless, the construction of large centres such as the *residencias sanitarias* and the *ciudades sanitarias* as a result of public insurance increased the weighting of hospital beds available in the public sector compared with the private sector (Table 1.5). However, it is necessary to be aware of the limitations of these figures. In this regard, an article published in the *El País* newspaper in 1977 pointed out that 'the national statistics in the Catalogue of Hospitals would lead to false conclusions. There are many centres with an extremely low occupation rate and others that should be closed. We have found numerous examples that do not meet minimum standards either technically or in terms of comfort'.[58] There was still a long way to go within an exceptionally turbulent political context (lack of leadership at the national level) and social conflict (strikes and protests) and in the middle of the country's transition to democracy after almost forty years of dictatorship.[59] The 1970 Foessa Report revealed that Spain had one of the most deficient hospital situations in Europe.

Table 1.5: Hospitals and beds in Spain according to property ownership

Year	Public		Private		Total	
	Hospitals	Beds	Hospitals	Beds	Hospitals	Beds
1949	737	89,079	885	38,264	1622	127,343
1963	589	102,250	1037	52,036	1226	154,286
1973	488	125,254	797	55,293	1285	180,547
1977	476	132,907	753	61,190	1229	194,097
1981	409	130,298	645	63,598	1054	193,896
1986	380	116,938	509	54,922	889	171,860

Source: See Table 4 and for 1973, 1977 and 1986, see *Estadística de Establecimientos Sanitarios con Régimen de Internado*, web INE (1978), AEE (1980), 349 and (1990), 118. Source 1981: Statistical Yearbook of Spain (*Anuario Estadístico de España*), 1985, 709.

The exclusion of insurance companies and mutuals from the private management of the SOE after the implementation of the Basic Law of Social Security of 1963 did not result in the decline of private hospitals. They actually flourished on the basis of agreements to provide beds for surgery patients who were insured under the SOE, along with the demand for private hospitals to cover certain specialities, especially gynaecological, and for the provision of medical attention to an emerging middle class and public servants with privileged mutual coverage. Although there are no public data on the number of agreements between private sector hospitals and the Social Security (former INP and SGM hospitals, see Table 1.4), the *Anuario Financiero y de Sociedades Anónimas* yearbook for 1980, with data from 1964 to 1980, includes the creation of joint-stock companies in the hospital sector, especially in Madrid (15) and to a lesser extent in Barcelona (5) and Biscay (4). This coincides with the demand for hospital care linked to urban growth, increased incomes and a shortage of beds. As a result of these factors, the number of private beds grew continuously from 52,036 in 1963 to 63,598 in 1981. However, the number of hospitals belonging to the entire private sector was actually declining, falling from 1,037 to 645 in the same period (Table 1.5). The rise in the number of beds was due to the increase in the size of hospitals, a similar trend to the evolution of public hospitals. This process was linked to the closure and removal from the catalogue of establishments serving as refuges for the elderly, the closure of private establishments where there was little activity and also the grouping and re-categorisation of hospitals and medical centres that were previously accounted for independently. Within this group of private hospitals, comprising companies operating for profit but also the Church, the Spanish Red Cross and private charitable or voluntary hospitals, the latter continued to benefit from favourable tax treatment and were exempt from paying taxes imposed on the assets of legal persons. This was despite the fact that the number of pay beds was progressively increasing, which demonstrated that they were also engaged in profit-making activities.[60]

By the end of the dictatorship, the problems of the health system in general and the hospital system in particular continued to be very similar to those observed in the previous section. It is nevertheless true that the percentage of the population covered had increased, provision had been extended and there were more *residencias sanitarias*. Moreover, these public hospitals had improved with respect to private hospitals in terms of facilities and resources and had introduced new training methods for specialised medical staff. However, health care continued in the hands of the INP, an institute that managed the Social Security accounts in an opaque fashion and which had a long history of corruption, and the hospital system remained fragmented, without coordination, and with serious deficiencies in its internal functioning. The poor territorial distribution of hospitals had led to an unequal allocation of material and human resources (Table 1.6).[61] In general, the country lacked a health strategy in a framework where there was neither a Ministry of Health nor a general health law to define the model to follow. *Residencias Sanitarias* and *Ciudades Sanitarias* continued to specialise in acute medicine and surgical operations, within a structure where public and private hospitals coexisted and collaborated in a number of ways.

When Franco died in November 1975, Spain had not recognised health care as a basic right, the SOE was far from achieving universal coverage (1975: 61.74%),[62] its provisions remained limited, its accounts had serious financial imbalances. There was no health law that defined the country's health care model and no Ministry of Health to manage the country's health policy in a coordinated and structured manner. Almost forty years of dictatorship had left too many tasks pending in the health sphere. Nonetheless, in 1981, on the verge of passing legislation to tackle these shortcomings, the public hospital system in Spain was actually evolving better than the private hospital sector, although it still required the collaboration of private hospitals (Table 1.4).

Table 1.6: Public and private hospital facilities in 1977 (Number)

Facilities	Social Security hospitals*	Private hospitals
Operating theatre	100	93
X-rays	96	80
Pharmacy	87	28
Emergency service	85	52
Laboratory	78	28
Radiotherapy	72	27
Blood bank	72	18
Intensive care unit	61	14
Artificial kidney machine	39	4
Cobalt bomb	24	2

Source: INP (Instituto Nacional de Previsión), *Investigación sobre la asistencia farmacéutica en España: Estudio socioeconómico sobre el conjunto de la asistencia sanitaria española* (Madrid: Ministerio de Trabajo, 1977), 285-306. *This basically refers to INP (*Residencias Sanitarias, Ciudades Sanitarias*), and SGM hospitals, see Table 4.

On reflection: democracy, universal coverage and decentralisation of health care in Spain

The establishment of democracy in Spain enabled some key foundations to be laid for the development of the country's health care model. In 1977, Fernández Ordoñez's eagerly-awaited tax reform, which modernised the Spanish fiscal system, was approved. In the same year, it was agreed that the state contribution to financing Social Security would be progressively increased to 20 per cent of its budget. In 1981, this contribution was set at just 10.39% of the total revenue of the system, and the contribution of employers and employees was 73.85% and 13.14% of the revenue budget, respectively. Meanwhile, also in 1977, the INP (plagued by corruption and blighted by the opacity of its accounts) disappeared and a new institution was created for the administration and management of health care services, the INSALUD (*Instituto Nacional de Salud*; National Health Institute).[63] In parallel, during the first legislature of the democracy, the Ministry of Health was created (1977), which integrated all competencies in health matters, managed up to this point by the Ministry of the Interior, and the competencies of the Under-Secretariat for Social Security. The foundations for change had been set in place, but Spain still lacked a general law establishing a health and hospital system. The first governments of the democracy, from 1977 to 1985, were incapable of successfully implementing the project due to the lack of political consensus. Something similar occurred with the private health care sector, which during the years of the transition to democracy was awaiting necessary reforms to modernise both its regulatory framework and its business structure.

After years of debate on the health model since the beginning of the transition to democracy and no consensual solution, PSOE's victory with an absolute majority in the elections of 1982 opened the way to the success of the health bill in Congress. In presenting the bill to Parliament in 1985, the Health Minister Ernest Lluch indicated that his project proposed the universalisation of provision (to meet social demand) and the creation of more employment in the health sector, free exercise of the medical profession (doctors who worked in public hospitals could also open private clinics) and an improvement in working conditions (a demand of unions and professional groups). Finally, in his speech the Minister pointed out that, in fact, 'it was not possible to establish a National Health Service' in Spain, as there existed a system allowing for 'political autonomy of services', although the state must provide minimum guarantees for all Spaniards (a demand of the autonomous communities—*comunidades autónomas*—that is, regional governments). Furthermore, the project proposed the 'maintenance of a mixed funding mechanism where social contributions continue to be considered as a source of funding', although with the intention to progressively increase the state's contribution. The passage of the bill encountered the opposition of conservative party (AP/PP)[64] and communist party (PCE), although from very different perspectives and strategies. The only consensus of all the groups seemed to be on the need for a health care reform and on the serious (financial, managerial and health care provision) problems of the Spanish health system.

After a stormy process of more than three years, with complicated negotiations among diverse political sectors, social forces and professional groups, the General Health Law was passed in 1986. It addressed the difficult task of laying the foundations for two complex processes:[65] the modernisation of Spanish health care and the decentralisation of its management. However, the text failed to satisfy almost anyone. The political right labelled the law as '*dirigista*' (dirigiste) and basically accused it of not establishing the free choice of doctor and health system.[66] Progressive sectors criticised the law for not setting up a national health service, along the lines of the British model, and for not guaranteeing that health care be provided totally free of charge (limited care benefits in some medical specialties) and, consequently, its universality. After numerous debates, adjustments, and a lack of consensus, the law, *Ley General de Sanidad (LGS) 14/1986, of 25 April*, was finally passed with the votes in favour of left-wing parties (PSOE and PCE) and Basque and Catalan nationalist parties (PNV and CIU),[67] which entailed the state legislative implementation of the right to health protection established in the Spanish Constitution. However, the text of this law contained more a set of principles and far-reaching goals than a plan for the immediate implementation of health reform.[68]

Meanwhile, the processes for the transfer of health care management to the autonomous communities had already begun, which by 1986 had now been assigned fifty-four hospitals with 14,604 inpatient units. The transfer of functions and services to the autonomous communities was initiated in 1981 with Catalonia and was concluded in 2001. The profound changes that Spanish health care underwent during this period with the passage of a health law, the process of transferring health care to the autonomous communities, the transformation of the hospital map and the modernisation of health and hospital services did not break the link between the public and private hospital sectors. Ernest Lluch stated during the debate on the health law in Congress that his project aspired to 'maintain a stable relationship between public and private health care' within the public sector's guidelines (demand of the private sector).[69] Moreover, he added that 'most of the private hospital sector in this country operates in relation to the public sector. In other words, it could not survive without having interaction with the public sector'. According to his calculations, only seventeen per cent of private health services were not part of agreements with the public sector. These services were used by high income groups. These words proved to be true, and during this period public and private hospital sectors continued to be closely linked.

Furthermore, the oil crises of the 1970s, the increase of the bed capacity of the public system and the consequent reduction in agreements signed with the private sector, along with the obsolete facilities of some small hospitals, triggered a crisis in the private hospital system. This was the case in Bilbao where, in 1984, the INSALUD rescinded the agreements of eleven small and medium-sized clinics.[70] This phenomenon was instrumental in the fact that the number of private hospitals fell again from 645 in 1981 to 509 in 1986 and the number of beds went from 63,598 to 54,092 (Table 1.5).

The private sector implemented numerous strategies to resist this downturn. Three of them are worth highlighting: the creation of associations of private hospitals and lobbies,[71] the need to modernise in order to meet the demand of civil servants' mutuals,[72] and the regional decentralisation of health care were the mechanisms that made it possible to overcome the crisis and reinforce the private system in the following decades.[73] With the devolution of health care competencies to the autonomous communities and the adoption of models closer to the interests of the private sector in some regions, the private hospital sector started to grow again. This growth was once again sustained by agreements with public health services, and some regional governments even handed over the management of public hospitals to private companies.

In conclusion, the originality of the Spanish public health model was determined by the long Franco dictatorship that made the adoption of a welfare state impossible, without a structural and financing model defined at the beginning, although some Bismarckian elements were incorporated to support the compulsory health insurance programme within a social contribution system. The long transition to democracy generated an in-depth debate over the health system model. Finally, a model financed in large part by the state (following the British model) was presented but opposing positions among political parties only allowed the passage of a Health Law. This law, although it progressively increased the financing of the state funding through taxes, did not manage to introduce universal coverage and benefits. In addition, its approval in 1986 went against the current of neoliberal policy processes that were underway in many European countries, imposing cuts in social spending, especially in public health systems. On the other hand, for pragmatic, financial and ideological reasons, the first state interventions under the Franco dictatorship when health insurance was created in 1942 had the opened way to the active collaboration of insurance companies and private hospitals insurance benefits.

The transfer of health care competencies to autonomous communities from the 1980s consolidated the public health model in many territories, especially those governed by left-wing parties, which put an end to signing of agreements with the private sector for the provision of health services. In other regions, especially those governed by conservative parties, health care management was encouraged in collaboration with private insurance and hospital companies. The key historical factors that determined the evolution of public and private health care derived from the state health model were both basically political (dictatorship and democracy) and financial (a regressive tax system until 1977). The dictatorship, for reasons of propaganda and ideology, delayed the adoption of health insurance that could be considered as part of a welfare state model. The lack of consensus in the first ten years of the transition to democracy prolonged this situation. Despite this, the Spanish health system managed to reach the top positions in the international health rankings by the end of the twentieth century. Public investment during democracy and the training of excellent professionals in the field of health care played a key role in this success. It may well be the case that this could have been achieved much earlier if the country had enjoyed democratic institutions similar to those of other Western European countries after the Second World War.

1. Both authors gratefully acknowledge financial support from the European Union, the European Regional Development Fund (ERDF), and Spain's Ministry of Science and Innovation—State Research Agency—for the project entitled "The historical keys of hospital development in Spain and its international comparison during the twentieth century", ref. RTI2018-094676-B-I00.
* Corresponding Author. Email: mvilar@udc.es. Postal address: Margarita Vilar-Rodríguez; Facultad de Economía y Empresa, Universidad de A Coruña, Campus de Elviña, s/n, 15071 A Coruña (Spain).

2. Bernard Harris and Paul Bridgen (eds), Charity and Mutual Aid in Europe and North America since 1800 (New York: Routledge, 2007); Bernard Harris, The Origins of the British Welfare State: State and Social Welfare in England and Wales, 1800–1945 (Basingstoke: Palgrave Macmillan, 2004).

3. David Rosner, A Once Charitable Enterprise: Hospitals and Health Care in Brooklyn and New York, 1885–1915 (New York: Cambridge University Press, 1982); Rosemary Stevens, In Sickness and in Wealth: American Hospitals in the Twentieth Century (New York: Basic Books, 1989); Martin Gorsky and Sally Sheard (eds), Financing Medicine: The British Experience since 1750 (London and New York: Routledge, 2006); Steven Cherry, 'Before the National Health Service: Financing the Voluntary Hospitals, 1900-1939', Economic History Review, 50, 305-26 (1997); Martin Gorsky, John Mohan and Martin Powell, 'The financial health of voluntary hospitals in interwar Britain', Economic History Review, 55, 533–57. Pierre-Yves Domin, Une histoire économique de l'hôpital (XIXe-XXe siècles). Une analyse rétrospective du développement hospitalier, Tome I (1803-1945) (Paris: Comité d'histoire Sécurité Social, 2008).

4. Melissa A. Thomasson, 'From Sickness to Health: The Twentieth-Century Development of the Demand for Health Insurance', The Journal of Economic History, 60, 2 (2000), 504–508; Christy F. Chapin, Ensuring America's Health (New York: Cambridge University Press, 2015); John E. Murray, Origins of American Health Insurance: A History of Industrial Sickness Funds (New York: Yale University Press, 2007).

5. Stevens, op. cit. (note 3).

6. For more information on the transformations in private health insurance in recent decade, see Sarah Thomson and Elias Mossialos, Private health insurance in the European Union. Final report prepared for the European Commission, Directorate General for Employment, Social Affairs and Equal Opportunities (London: LSE Health and Social Care, London School of Economics and Political Science, 2009); as well as Patrick Hassenteufel and Bruno Palier, 'Towards Neo-Bismarckian Health Care States? Comparing Health Insurance Reforms in Bismarckian Welfare Systems', in Bruno Palier and Claude Martin (eds), In Reforming the Bismarckian Welfare Systems, (Malden: Willey-Blackwell, 2008), 40-61; Laura Cabiedes and Ana Guillén, 'Adopting and Adapting Managed Competition: Health Care Reform in Southern Europe', Social Science & Medicine, 52 (2001), 1205–17; Elias Mossialos and Sara Allin, 'Interest groups and health system reform in Greece', West European Politics, 28, 2 (2005), 421-45; Rebeca Jasso-Aguilar, Howard Waitzkin and Angela

Landwehr, 'Multinational Corporations and Health Care in the United States and Latin America: Strategies, Actions, and Effects', Journal of Health and Social Behavior, 45 (2004), 136-57.

7. See, for example, Gerard A. Ritter, El Estado Social, su origen y desarrollo en una comparación internacional (Madrid: Ministerio de Trabajo, 1991); Thomas Janoski and Alexander M. Hicks (eds), The Comparative Political Economy of the Welfare State (Cambridge: Cambridge University Press, 1994), 254-77; Isabela Mares, The Politics of Social Risk. Business and Welfare State Development (Cambridge: Cambridge University Press, 2003); David M. Cutler and Richard Johnson, 'The Birth and Growth of the Social Insurance State: Explaining Old Age and Medical Insurance across countries', Public Choice, 120 (2004), 87-121.

8. Diputaciones were provincial government institutions created from 1812 onward, see Ana M. Rodríguez Martín, 'La participación femenina en la Beneficencia española. La Junta de damas de la casa de maternidad expósitos de Barcelona, 1853-1903', Cuestiones de Igualdad y la diferencia, 9 (2013), 134-57.

9. This criteria is the same as that used for Margarita Vilar-Rodríguez and Jerònia Pons-Pons, 'Competition and collaboration between public and private sectors: the historical construction of the Spanish hospital system, 1942–86', The Economic History Review, 72 (2019), 1384-1408.

10. Pedro Carasa Soto, El sistema hospitalario español en el siglo XIX. De la asistencia benéfica al modelo sanitario actual (Valladolid: Universidad de Valladolid, 1985),

30-4. Josep M Comelles; Elisa Alegre-Agís and Josep Barceló-Prats, 'Del hospital de pobres a la cultura hospitalo-céntrica. Economía política y cambio cultural en el sistema hospitalario catalán', Kamchatka. Revista de Análisis Cultural, 10 (2017), 57-85; Margarita Vilar-Rodríguez and Jerònia Pons Pons, 'The long shadow of charity in the Spanish hospital system, c. 1870-1942', Social History, 44, 3 (2019), 317-42.

11. This process obliged the sale of property belonging to religious corporations and the closure of many monasteries, convents, colleges and religious communities, which put an end to their tithes and other incomes. The disentailment laws cut off the sources of financing of religious charitable establishments. Consequently, some religious hospitals were destined for public use and came under the control of civil authorities, above all municipal or provincial councils. See Josep Fontana, Crisis del Antiguo Régimen 1808-1833 (Barcelona: Critica, 1979).

12. Mariano Esteban de Vega, 'La asistencia liberal española, beneficencia pública y previsión particular', Historia Social, XIII (1992), 123-8.

13. For the Basque case, see Pedro M. Pérez Castroviejo, 'La formación del sistema hospitalario vasco administración y gestión económica, 1800-1936', TST: Transportes, Servicios y telecomunicaciones, 3-4 (2002), 73-97. For Málaga, see the documentation deposited in the Diputación (Provincial Council) Archive, link: www.malaga.es/base/descargas/.../breve-historia-fondo-documental-hospital-civil (accessed 26 November 2018).

14. Ministerio de Gobernación, Apuntes para el estudio y la organización en España de las instituciones de beneficencia y previsión. Memoria de la Dirección General de Administración (Madrid: Establecimientos Tip. Sucesores de Rivadeneyra, impresores de la Casa Real, 1909), CI-CII and LXIV); Elena Maza, 'El mutualismo en España, 1900-1941. Ajustes e interferencias', in Santiago Castillo and Rafael Ruzafa (eds), La previsión social en la historia (Madrid: Siglo XXI, 2009), 333-68.

15. Statistical Yearbook of Spain (Anuario Estadístico de España) (1859-1860), 151, 160.

16. Ministerio de Gobernación, op. cit. (note 14), CI-CII and LXIV; and Maza, op. cit. (note 14), 336.

17. Using the population data of the National Statistics Institute (Instituto Nacional de Estadística, INE) for Spain in 1910, of 19,990,000 inhabitants (link: www.ine.es).

18. This certificate was required, for example, in the Hospital Hidrológico de Carlos III in Trillo in order to receive medicinal baths. Moreover, the document was supposed to indicate whether the poor sick person was in receipt of aid from any charitable association or corporation and, if so, how much. Gazeta de Madrid, no. 182, 1 July 1883, 2.

19. Ministerio de Gobernación, op. cit. (note 14), CI-CII and LXIV; and Maza, op. cit. (note 14), 336.

20. Gazeta de Madrid, no. 45, 12 February 1879.

21. Notably, among others, the decree of 27 April 1875 and another specific law of 14 March 1899.

22. Gazeta de Madrid no. 51, 20 February 1876, 429.

23. See for example the exemptions granted in the Gazeta de Madrid no. 106, 16 April 1913, 147; and Gazeta de Madrid no. 234, 21 August 1920.

24. One example would be the authorisation of the Directorate General for Taxation (Dirección General de Tributos) for a charity raffle between 28 April and 29 May 1963 for a total of 400,000 tickets costing 2.5 pesetas each, Boletín Oficial del Estado, BOE (Official State Gazette) no. 96, 22 April 1963, 6718.

25. Vicente Pérez Moreda, David-Sven Reher and Alberto Sanz Gimeno, La conquista de la salud: mortalidad y modernización en la España contemporánea (Madrid: Marcial Pons Historia, 2015).

26. Biblioteca Nacional de España (Spanish National Library), Fondos históricos digitalizados, Reseña del primer ejercicio del Instituto de Terapéutica Operatoria del Hospital de la Princesa (Madrid, 1881).

27. Pérez Moreda, Reher and Sanz, op. cit. (note 25). Madrid is described as the 'city of death' for this reason in Isabel Porras, 'Un acercamiento a la situación higiénico—sanitaria de los distritos de Madrid en el tránsito del siglo XIX al XX', Asclepio, Revista de historia de la medicina y de la ciencia, 54, 1 (2002), 219-51.

28. Marcel.lí Moreta i Amat, Cataluña en el movimiento mutualista de previsión

social en España (Barcelona: unpublished manuscript, 1991), 69; Jerònia Pons Pons and Margarita Vilar-Rodríguez, 'Friendly Societies, Commercial Insurance, and the State in Sickness Risk Coverage, The Case of Spain (1880-1944)', International Review of Social History, 56 (2011), 71-101.

29. Jerònia Pons-Pons and Margarita Vilar-Rodríguez, El seguro de salud privado y público en España. Su análisis en perspectiva histórica (Zaragoza: Prensas de la Universidad de Zaragoza, 2014), 153.

30. Angel P. Martínez Soto and Miguel A. Pérez de Perceval, 'Asistencia sanitaria en la minería de la Sierra de Cartagena/La Unión (1850/1914)', Revista de la Historia de la Economía y de la Empresa, IV (2010), 93-124.

31. The causes of this backwardness can be found in the political apathy during the Primo de Rivera dictatorship and in the financial difficulties for implementation, see Francisco Comín, Historia de la Hacienda Pública II. España (1808-1995) (Barcelona: Crítica, 1996) vol II, 272. In addition, insurance companies and doctors opposed the implantation method, see Josefina Cuesta, Los seguros sociales en la España del siglo XX. Las crisis de la Restauración (Madrid: Ministerio de Trabajo y Seguridad Social, 1988), 415.

32. Vilar-Rodríguez and Pons-Pons, op. cit. (note 9).

33. For more on the hospital coverage of the two armies in conflict, see Jose M. Gómez Teruel, La hospitalización en Sevilla a través de los tiempos (Sevilla: Fundación Real Colegio de Médicos de Sevilla, 2006).

34. National Catholicism was the state consent that the Franco regime gave to the Catholic Church, as an institution legitimising the dictatorship, so that it could exercise control of decisive social and political spaces. Public morals, social behaviour, education and charity were subject to the authority and ecclesiastical norms of the Catholic hierarchy, see Carme Molinero, La captación de las masas política social y propaganda en el régimen franquista (Madrid: Cátedra, 2005).

35. The state did not contribute any money to the implementation of the SOE. 50 million pesetas of this period, coming from the funds of other social insurance schemes and family allowances, were used. Henceforth, the sickness insurance was sustained with the social contributions of workers (above all) and employers, in a context of precarious working and wage conditions, and recourse to the issue of public debt and credit from the Bank of Spain. Boletín de Información del Instituto Nacional de Previsión, 1944, no. 6, 853. This financing plan was foreshadowed in the Law of 1942, BOE 27 December 1942, 10592-97, art. 38.

36. For more on the health coverage of the agricultural population in Spain, see Margarita Vilar-Rodríguez and Jerònia Pons-Pons, 'La cobertura social de los trabajadores en el campo español durante la dictadura franquista', Historia Agraria, 66 (2015), 177-210.

37. Boletín de Información del Instituto Nacional de Previsión, 1944-1945; Revista Española de Seguridad Social, 1947-1951; Anuario Estadístico de España, 1950, 1955, 1960 and 1963.

38. See Margarita Vilar-Rodríguez and Jerònia Pons-Pons (eds.), Un Siglo de Hospitales entre lo público y lo privado (1886-1986) (Madrid: Marcial Pons, 2018), 226.

39. Carme Pérez, 'El misterio acceso a la gestión sanitaria', El Español newspaper, 3 February 2014, link: https://cronicaglobal.elespanol.com/pensamiento/el-misterioso-acceso-a-la-gestion-sanitaria_4526_102.html

40. The Residences or Sanitary Cities were built by the National Institute of Housing (Instituto Nacional de la Vivienda). See, for example, that of Valencia built in 1967. Decreto 2299/1967, 19 August, BOE, n. 224, 19 September 1967, 12967-8.

41. For more on these hospitals, see Jacint Corbella, 'Cent anys de medicina. La nova facultat i l'Hospital Clínic de Barcelona 1906-2006', Catálogo de la Exposición Cent anys de Medicina. La nova Facultat i l'Hospital Clínic de Barcelona 1906-2006 (Barcelona: Digitised, online, 2006), link: http://diposit.ub.edu/dspace/handle/2445/33946.

42. For more on the military hospitals, see Pablo Gutiérrez, 'Los hospitales militares y la sanidad militar. La transición de un modelo segregado a la creación del ISFAS (1940-1986)' in Vilar-Rodríguez and Pons-Pons, op. cit. (note 38), 367-400.

43. The particular features of the Church's centres can be found in Pilar León, 'Hospitales de la Iglesia Católica en España', in Vilar-Rodríguez and Pons-Pons, op. cit. (note 38), 325-66. In countries such as Ireland, see Donnacha Lucey, The End of the Irish Poor Law? Welfare and healthcare reform in Revolutionary and Independent Ireland (Manchester: Manchester University Press, 2015), and in France the Church was influential in the creation of the hospital system, see Timothy B. Smith, 'The Social transformation of Hospitals and the Rise of Medical Insurance France, 1914-1943', The Historical Journal, XLI, 4 (1998), 1055-87.

44. Jerònia Pons-Pons and Margarita Vilar-Rodríguez, 'Labour repression and social justice in Franco's Spain: the political objectives of compulsory sickness insurance (1942-1957)', Labor History, 53, 2 (2012), 245-67.

45. Pons-Pons and Vilar-Rodríguez, op. cit. (note 29), 219.

46. Rafael Aracil, Sistema Gráfico de información sanitaria en España (Madrid, MSD-Artusa, 1996).

47. Not even the law on funding entitled Ley de Financiación y Perfeccionamiento de la Acción Protectora del Régimen General de la Seguridad Social, passed in 1972, achieved its main objective of correcting the imbalances in the system's accounts. BOE, 22 June 1972, no. 149, 11174.

48. The idea for these came from the monoblock hospital in USA, Beaujon Hospital in Paris, France, and Mayor Hospital in Milan, Italy. For more information, see Alberto Pieltain, 'Los hospitales de Franco. La versión autóctona de una arquitectura moderna', (Unpub. Ph.D. Dissertation at Universidad Politécnica of Madrid, 2004), 257.

49. Josep Barceló and Josep M. Comelles, 'Las bases ideológicas del dispositivo hos-

pitalario en España: cambios y resistencias', in Vilar-Rodríguez and Pons-Pons, op. cit., (note 38), 83-138.

50. For more information, see Pons and Vilar, op. cit., (note 29), 239.

51. For further details, see the excellent work by Juli Nadal, La construcción de un éxito. Así se hizo nuestra sanidad pública (Barcelona: Ediciones La Lluvia, 2016), 60.

52. For further details, see Juan D. Tutosaus, Jesús Morán-Barriosa, and Fernando Pérez Iglesias, 'Historia de la formación sanitaria especializada en España y sus claves docentes', Educación Médica (2017), link: http://dx.doi.org/10.1016/j.edumed.2017.03.023.

53. Obtained from Jesús De Miguel Rodríguez, La reforma sanitaria en España. El capital humano en el sector sanitario (Madrid: Cambio 16, 1976), 198.

54. Order of 5 December 1967, BOE, no. 300, 16 December 1967, no. 300, 17456.

55. An observation already made by Luis Albertí López, 'La asistencia sanitaria en el conjunto de la previsión social española', in Varios autores (eds), 4 siglos de Acción Social, de la beneficencia al bienestar social, Seminario de historia de la acción social (Madrid: Siglo XXI, 1988), 297-338.

56. During the years 1972, 1973 and 1974, around 12,000 posts for doctors in the hospital system were filled by open competition on the basis of merit, most of them by doctors coming from the training programme for medical specialists (MIR), see Varios autores (eds), op. cit. (note 55), 333.

57. Pons-Pons and Vilar-Rodríguez, op. cit. (note 29), 137.

58. 'Reportaje: Los hospitales en España y la Seguridad Social/y 2', El País newspaper, link: https://elpais.com/diario/1977/08/17/sociedad/240616801_850215.html

59. Fernando J. Gallego, El mito de la transición. La crisis del franquismo y los orígenes de la democracia (1973-1977) (Barcelona: Crítica, 2008).

60. For example, in the case of Hospital de la Santísima Trinidad in Salamanca there were 121 charitable beds and 74 pay beds. The patrons of the hospital argued in favour of maintaining the proprietary category of private charitable hospital because the income from the pay beds was used to cover the costs of the charitable beds. BOE, no. 28, 2 February 1966, 1252-3.

61. Instituto Nacional de Previsión, INP, Investigación sobre la asistencia farmacéutica en España: Estudio socioeconómico sobre el conjunto de la asistencia sanitaria española (Madrid: Ministerio de Trabajo, 1977), 765.

62. Memoria Estadística de la Seguridad Social, 1976; and population data from Roser Nicolau, 'Población, salud y actividad', in Albert Carreras and Xavier Tafunell (coord), Estadísticas históricas de España, siglos XIX y XX (Bilbao: Fundación BBVA, 2005), vol. 1, 79-154.

63. In Vilar-Rodríguez and Pons-Pons, op. cit. (note 38), 406. There is an in-depth anal-

ysis of the debate surrounding public and private health insurance in Spain from the political transition to the General Health Law (Ley General de Sanidad). It includes aspects such as the corruption and opacity that accompanied the history of the INP; the lack of agreement on the country's health care model and the problems to draw up a general health law that achieved the necessary consensus in the Spanish Parliament.

64. AP/PP: Alianza Popular/Partido Popular; PCE: Partido Comunista Español.

65. Juan Ventura Victoria, 'Organización y gestion de la atención sanitaria', in Informe Anual del Sistema Nacional de Salud 2003 (Madrid, Ministerio de Sanidad y Consumo-Observatorio SNS, 2003), 307-62, see, http://www.msps.es/organizacion/sns/planCalidadSNS/pdf/equidad/Informe_Anual_nexo_V.pdf.

66. 'Change under democracy has barely touched the structure of health care', El País newspaper, 10 June 1986.

67. PSOE: Partido Socialista Obrero Español; PCE: Partido Comunista Español; PNV: Partido Nacionalista Vasco; CIU: Convergencia i Unió.

68. Pons-Pons and Vilar-Rodríguez, op. cit. (note 29), 363.

69. Diario de Sesiones del Congreso de los Diputados, II Legislatura, 1985, no. 215, sesión plenaria no. 215, 9852-55.

70. La Vanguardia newspaper, 9 April 1984, 14. The representatives of these clinics criticised these agreements because INSALUD assigned them 3,795 pesetas per day to care for each patient who required surgery. The clinics claimed that the real cost was actually 5,813 pesetas per patient per day, which was needed to maintain the agreement, with an average stay of 8 days per patient. Moreover, they reproached INSALUD with charging 19,000 pesetas per bed per day in its centres.

71. With respect to associationism, there were at least two associations in the private sector at this time: Unió Catalana d'Hospitals with headquarters in Barcelona, created in 1975, and the Federación Nacional de Clínicas Privadas, of national scope and located in Madrid.

72. In the mid-1970s there were four important mutuals that covered public servants: MUFACE for civil servants, MUGEJU for the judicial administration, MUNPAL for civil servants in the Local Administration and ISFAS for coverage of the armed forces. The government allowed the public servants who were members of these mutuals to have private health coverage via agreements with insurance companies. In 1984, 90.4 per cent of the members of MUFACE (1.1 million) were covered by private health insurance companies, see Jerònia Pons-Pons and Margarita Vilar-Rodríguez, 'The genesis, growth and organisational changes of private health insurance companies in Spain (1915-2015)', Business History 61, 3 (2019), 558-79, link: http://dx.doi.org/10.1080/00076791.2017.1374371.

73. The first of the Autonomous Communities to obtain the transfer of competencies in the area of health care was Catalonia, through Royal Decree 1517/1981, of 8 July.

Chapter 2

Charity and Philanthropy in the History of Brazilian Hospitals —The experience of São Paulo Holy House of Mercy and São Paulo Hospital: an outline of historical continuity[1]

Ana Nemi
(Federal University of São Paulo)

Health care in the Portuguese Empire: a prologue

Portuguese houses of mercy were lay brotherhoods where health care provision was guided by Christian values, and priorities were set by the Crown in relation to the interest of a local elite.[2] The first of them was founded in Lisbon in 1498, and they subsequently spread across the Portuguese Empire. The new houses of mercy were expected to operate in the model of the Lisbon *Misericórdia*, and had to deal with local particularities and the resulting connection with the elite.[3] In spite of these specificities, though, houses of mercy enjoyed privileges of royal protection. Amid the religious wars of the sixteenth century, their statutes were negotiated within the scope of the Council of Trent (1545-1563), which reinforced their Christian/Catholic identities and their autonomy from bishoprics.[4] Furthermore, this autonomy and the royal sanction for the practice of charity and the collection of testamentary donations conferred on the houses of mercy a structural governance role in the maintenance of the Portuguese Empire, through the exercise of local power by colonial elites, despite the differences between colonial spaces.[5] In other words, the Portuguese Empire coordinated local powers that were autonomous to a greater or lesser extent, depending on the significance of the local economy for the Royal Treasury, and on possible connections between local elites and those at the centre of the Empire. In addition, the Christian/Catholic notion of charity, with its emphasis on the virtues of poverty, turned the assistance of the poor into a means of salvation for the rich. This took the form of alms-giving while alive and of last wills and testaments benefiting the houses of mercy in death.

The sources of income of houses of mercy for the practice of charity, and, therefore, for the health care of the poor, were not homogeneous. The collection of alms was the privilege and main activity of the houses of mercy. Those houses located in more affluent cities, however, had higher liquidity, since they were engaged in trade. They also owned more real property, as they were recipients of assets linked to services and of testamentary donations that could be publicly auctioned.

During the sixteenth and seventeenth centuries, through the intervention of the Portuguese monarchy, a trend of incorporating hospitals into houses of mercy emerged. Across Europe, and in Portugal in particular, a separation existed between places of hospitality for travelers and pilgrims, and those dedicated to the care of the sick. These latter were fundamental to the activities carried out by houses of mercy, which, for this reason, built infirmaries and hospitals throughout the Empire.

Members of the brotherhoods of mercy were divided into nobles and the 'officials', who, although not members of the nobility, were business people and merchants not engaged in manual labour. The brothers managed the finances and could therefore use resources for their own benefit in the form of loans. In general, brothers were also members of local city councils, and this explains the frequent loans brotherhoods and city councils extended to one another, as well as the difficulty in collecting from politically influential debtors.[6] The social capital attached to belonging to a house of mercy brought with it political power and the opportunity to manage privately resources collected for the practice of charity. Although such charity was private when it came to collecting and applying financial resources, it was also intended to be public in the fulfillment of its activities. These were listed in the Commitment of the Misericordia, the set of principles and regulations for the operation of the Lisbon House of Mercy, which also guided the colonial houses.[7]

The fact that houses of mercy owned property and had never been taxed to the same extent as other institutions of the Empire, was the object of an injunction by the Marquis of Pombal in the second half of the eighteenth century. At the time, amid the diffusion of Enlightenment thought, it was evident to the Cabinet of the Marquis and the enlightened elites that Portugal should open its markets and take real property out of mortmain, which preserved inalienable rights of ownership in the hands of corporate boards, such as houses of mercy. In this public debate, elites considered that these houses of mercy represented a hindrance to the circulation of goods and workers. The Law of Good Reason, of 18 August 1769, was intended to control the receipt of inheritances by houses of mercy and other brotherhoods.[8] It was urgent to strengthen the nation's workforce by 'improving hygienic, nutritional, pharmaceutical, and medical practices' and by reorganising hospitals and home medical care, a task that would also be carried out by houses of mercy.[9] It was a moment when the Christian/Catholic notion of charity would be harshly criticised in the Portuguese Empire. The same criticism had been emerging since the sixteenth and seventeenth centuries in other European countries, such as England, France, and the German principalities.[10]

The tutelage imposed by the Pombaline reforms coincided with a time of discredit for houses of mercy and contributed to curtailing their autonomy.[11] Such discredit, however, was insufficient to change the tax exemption privileges that had always characterised the practice of charity in the Portuguese Empire, which can be explained by the relevance of the assistance services they offered. Neither was it enough to alter the links between houses of mercy and the local powers through which they negotiated and symbolically shared political power, even when the elites intended to withdraw from the boards of directors of houses of mercy at the turn of the eighteenth to the nineteenth century.

As a result, with the establishment of new liberal regimes in the nineteenth century, houses of mercy would have to settle accounts with the new civil powers. They would, though, retain their Christian/Catholic values and their enormous capacity of negotiation with city councils and the state. For this reason, anchored in their social work, houses of mercy would be subjected to modest taxation. In Portugal, *misericórdias* would maintain their central role in providing relief and health care for the poor. In the imperial territories, however, the histories of the houses of mercy took multiple and diverse paths. Even in the great Empire that was taking shape in Brazil, the fifteen brotherhoods founded until 1750 would have different trajectories.[12] The case of the town of São Paulo will be addressed below.

The Brotherhood São Paulo Holy House of Mercy between the Colonial Period and the Brazilian Empire

The Brotherhood São Paulo Holy House of Mercy (São Paulo *Misericórdia*), thought to have been founded in the sixteenth century, grew along with the city.[13] This means that its greatest period of expansion occured in the second half of the nineteenth century, *pari passu* with the coffee economy, but also with the debates arising from the circulation of knowledge and people in the Atlantic.

In the eighteenth century, the city of São Paulo strengthened its position as a gateway to the inland territory, serving as a point of departure and a place where care could be provided both to travelers on their way to the gold mines and to soldiers serving the interests of the Crown and local governments. The small hospital of São Paulo *Misericórdia* was founded in 1714, but would only start operating in premises acquired for this purpose in 1749. It would be much requested as a military infirmary. Many São Paulo citizens enriched in the mines were members of the brotherhood and advocated the foundation and consolidation of the hospital. In their view, the Brotherhood should cover sick care expenses and take actions to collect almsgiving to support its activities.[14]

The Empire's houses of mercy initially enjoyed relative freedom to conduct their activities. Multiple petitions, though, were filed to the Crown by the São Paulo Misericórdia's Board of Directors requesting aid and privileges equal to those granted to the Lisbon *Misericórdia*, since the town, depleted by mining, was short on financial resources.[15] In the late eighteenth century, however, strong imperial interference was imposed by the Marquis of Pombal, which continued for two reigns after Dom José I.[16] This subjected houses of mercy to the sceptical oversight of the legislators of the time, who wanted to exert control over testamentary donations which were falling into mortmain, and thus depriving the Crown and the municipality of tax revenue.[17] At the same time, they could not forgo the private charity offered houses of mercy, since these alleviated social problems by means of their hospitals and foundling wheels.[18] In this sense, the Royal Charter of 18 October 1806, which obliged all the Empire's houses of mercy to abide by the Commitment of the Lisbon Misericordia, is emblematic of the centralisation processes taking place in the Portuguese Empire and of the attempts to control local autonomous institutions. The intention was to reorganise care provision by controlling what the Enlightenment called vagrancy and by setting workers apart from those who engaged in begging for unworthy reasons.[19]

It was also in this conjuncture that the *tropeiro*, who had succeeded the *sertanista*,[20] became a predecessor of the farmer who sought to take root in the lands of São Paulo plateau with sugar plantations and, still in their early stages, coffee plantations.[21] Thus São Paulo's modest elite faced an influx of soldiers, royal employees and travellers, and sought new ways to balance its plantation interests and local power with the Crown's injunctions—marked by the arrival of the Majorat of Mateus in 1765.[22] This small elite would combine the exercise of political power in the city council with the practice of charity in the brotherhood. This combination was maintained even in the face of the disruptions arising from the Napoleonic Wars, the coming of the Portuguese court to Brazil, and plans for the independence of Brazil.

Most studies of the brotherhoods of mercy in Portuguese America state that the property and resources of these institutions were derived from donations and bequests from individuals, as had occurred in Portugal. From what can be seen in their statutes, this was a structuring element of their activity.[23] Although São Paulo *Misericórdia* had fewer resources available to conduct its work, it availed itself of public resources and benefited from tax exemption privileges, just like other *misericórdias*.[24] However, at the turn of the nineteenth century, a hygienist discourse very much in line with the Enlightenment and civilising aspirations of the time, increasingly gained space in some political speeches at the São Paulo City Council. This set out medical justifications for organising the public and private spheres of citizens' lives. Such speeches indicated the path and shape that the State was taking, both locally and nationwide, towards a rational arrangement of the 'turba'—the common people. They represented the limited place of Enlightenment thought that coexisted with police action and with the violence immanent in a slaveholding and unequal society.[25] The implementers of the new politics that emanated from the 1806 Royal Charter were primarily landowners who took back control of the Brotherhood's Board of Directors before the proclamation of Brazilian independence in 1822, due to their dissatisfaction with the Crown's protégés brought in by the Majorat of Mateus.

It was in this context that São Paulo expanded the political and social domain of its house of mercy, which retained its privileges and its role in the development of new precepts aimed at reorganising the hygiene and health practices of São Paulo's citizens. It is possible, therefore, to observe a redesignation of houses of mercy in the Portuguese Atlantic, at once retaining their private origins but also relying on public resources and tax exemption privileges to practice private charity. This state of affairs was made possible by the political influence of colonial elites, which operated in those institutions through the nineteenth and twentieth centuries. After the independence of Brazil the established São Paulo *Misericórdia* elite constructed a building for its hospital in 1824. It then set out its ideals and powers in the Commitment of 1827, passed in 1836 by the São Paulo Provincial Assembly. At that time, the imbrication of the provincial assemblies of the Brazilian Empire, city councils, and houses of mercy was reflected in the composition of the directing boards of brotherhoods, which always included provincial deputies, councilmen, and landowners, configuring a legal and effective articulation between private elites and public powers.[26]

Throughout the nineteenth century, São Paulo *Misericórdia* would fund its activities with revenue derived from renting out its real estate. This had been obtained through bequests, from donations by the brothers and from public resources in the form of financial aid and tax exemptions, which were justified by its provision to the poor. Nevertheless, the brotherhood was always constrained by the economic and social condition of the city and province in which they were located. This model was also replicated for hospitals not linked to brotherhoods of mercy, which started to be called *filantrópicos*—philanthropic hospitals—in the late nineteenth century, and which also aimed to provide free health care to the poor. Márcia Barros Silva studied the nineteenth-century Annals of São Paulo Provincial Legislative Assembly and found multiple and diverse requests for health care funding from the São Paulo *Misericórdia* hospital.[27] She also found aid requests for the construction of other hospitals:

> 'Other aid requests were intended for the construction and maintenance of leprosariums and mental asylums. The requests were similar to those made by houses of mercy: allocation of direct funds, or creation of lotteries and other fundraising activities were deemed appropriate for this type of institution. These benefits, always insufficient, also had to compete with other solicitations for construction of medical accommodation. For example, in 1872, a project for the creation of a charity hospital in the city of São Paulo, which had been advanced by the physician J. F. dos Reis in the previous year, was rejected on the grounds that the Holy House was already providing health care in the city.' [28]

Thus, in the experience of São Paulo *Misericórdia*, it is possible to observe the maintenance of the exercise of private charity institutionalised in the Portuguese Empire, but now in a dialogue with public power that would become increasingly eloquent and effective throughout the nineteenth century. The development of both the city and the coffee economy in the late nineteenth century brought the arrival of immigrants and population growth, lending a new urgency to public health measures. In this context, some noteworthy sanitary measures included dealing with polluted water and 'miasmas', sewage treatment, collective vaccination, and regulation of hospitals and public areas. Another issue was the number of hospital beds, the demand for which increased at the same rate as the city and its population. This problem was worsened by the fact that the São Paulo *Misericórdia* also received patients from other cities of the province. It was not by chance that the Republic, established in 1889, would witness a rise in the number of philanthropic hospitals. The health care provided by houses of mercy was already lacking, and these new hospitals would develop on the same basis established by *misericórdias*: private charity with public funding delivered in distinct ways and in dialogue with local and state public powers.[29]

How did this compare with developments elsewhere? A debate about the advantages of the new philanthropy over older endowed charity had also occurred in eighteenth- and nineteenth-century England, leading to a different rationale for philanthropy. The voluntary hospital institutions established subsequently reduced considerably their level of generosity towards poor people deemed healthy and able for work. Their premise was that philanthropic actions should be guided by the strengthening of the nation's workforce and by their social usefulness rather than by piety. It called for less reliance on individual donors and for greater continuity and for more consistent and effective funding mechanisms.[30] England then developed a two-sided model: one with public institutions funded with tax revenue from the local poor rates; the other with philanthropic institutions that benefited from tax exemptions and whose trustees defined the remit, locations, and the medical practices deemed appropriate. On the American side of the Atlantic, the thirteen British colonies replicated this model, maintaining it after independence, even considering a greater presence of the community in the business of local charity.[31]

In nineteenth-century Portugal meanwhile, the Crown exerted strong influence over the administration of houses of mercy, with debate and legislation proposing health measures in the nation's general interest. Despite this, however, the organisation of hospitals remained characterised by Christian charity, whereby private donations by God-fearing citizens were expected to be sufficient to fund these institutions. Such was the case of the most important hospital of the Lisbon *Misericórdia*, São José Hospital, whose directors complained and denounced the insufficiency and irregularity of allocated resources.[32]

However, in the town of São Paulo, the penetration of new ideas from the Enlightenment was not sufficient to subvert the older traditions and mentalities of Christian/Catholic charity in the health care provided by São Paulo *Misericórdia* hospital. Only the Republic would show some vigor in doing so.

Charity and Philanthropy in the Republican Period

In Brazil, it was in the Republican period that the progress of public health actions that claimed to be philanthropic became manifest, especially in the creation of new hospitals.[33] The federal law No. 173, of 10 December 1893, proposed the regulation of associations created for moral, religious, artistic, scientific, political, and recreational purposes, thus laying down the criteria for the foundation of a plurality of non-profit civil associations with diverse interests. The *filantrópicos* were dedicated to providing health care services, and were most often set up by physicians or groups of physicians. These are the ones addressed in this study.[34] The Republic, therefore, found a legal manner to maintain the institutional arrangement that secured for houses of mercy and other philanthropic institutions the right to use both private and public resources to provide health care and build new premises when needed. The statutory characterisation of a civil association as not-for-profit entailed the possibility of exemption from certain taxes. In the same way, the provision of public health services and free hospital beds to the poor entailed the possibility of applying for public resources. These resources would come in the form of extraordinary revenue or, more commonly from the 1930s on, in the form of subventions approved by federal, state, and municipal assemblies.[35]

The aforementioned federal law No. 173, therefore, gave legal status to a practice that had been developing in the negotiations that led to the construction of the new São Paulo *Misericórdia* hospital, opened in 1884. Reports by Treasury officials pointed to the need for expanding the hospital due to an increase in demand for medical care in the city. Coffee farmers, who were for the most part brothers of São Paulo *Misericórdia*, made contributions and donations for the new building. These same brothers competed for the opportunity to donate the land for its construction, seeking to make the location of their stores and businesses more valuable. Once the hospital and its modern facilities were declared open, the negotiations with federal, state and municipal governments to fund the hospital's services began.[36]

At São Paulo *Misericórdia*, there was an extraordinary increase in revenue coming from public resources, in comparison with ordinary resources (rents, lotteries, donations by brothers etc.) throughout the nineteenth century and into the early twentieth century. This can be verified by cross-checking the reports presented by the Brotherhood and the debates recorded in the Annals of the Provincial Assembly (after 1889, State Assembly) and the São Paulo City Council. This characteristic would be replicated in the new *filantrópicos*. A public health model was, therefore, being consolidated in which public resources were employed by non-profit private institutions that defined their area of activity and the health care practices to be offered. It should also be noted that this political choice, negotiated by the economic and intellectual elites, resulted in a reduction of public funds obtained through the tax exemptions that such civil associations received due to their non-profit status. Physicians were the most active members of the intellectual elite, keen to influence the paths of public health and the individual medical assistance provided in hospitals.

The framework of Brazilian hospital philanthropy was one in which private institutions fulfilled public purposes in return for tax relief and light regulation. This provided physicians with considerable encouragment to submit proposals for sanitary schemes and new hospital foundations to the public authorities. From the standpoint of collective action, the Republic's first decades were marked by campaigns that aimed to regulate housing, ports, stores, factories, water distribution, sewage treatment, landfill sites and cemetries, as well as to implement large-scale vaccination, all in an attempt to develop salubrious and civilised sanitary practices. Individual medical assistance would only become a matter of concern in the 1920s, when social security medicine took its first steps.[37] The regulation and construction of new hospitals would, therefore, conform to the inheritance and tradition of houses of mercy on the one hand, and with physicians' interests and ideology on the other. Therefore, between the late nineteenth and the early twentieth centuries, the construction of new *filantrópicos* was accompanied by debates concerning the connections between mental illness and criminology. In the city of São Paulo, for example, this trend was typified by Juquery Mental Asylum, founded in 1898, and Pinel Sanatorium, founded in 1929, both of which were the result of projects advanced by physicians.[38] Individual, inpatient and outpatient care for the poor was still largely reliant on houses of mercy, since more affluent classes benefited from private medical care. The 1930s, however, would bring changes to individual medical assistance, and the experience at the São Paulo Hospital is quite illustrative of them.

São Paulo School of Medicine Civil Association and São Paulo Hospital

In 1933, a group of thirty-three physicians founded São Paulo School of Medicine Civil Association (SPSM). Its 'non-profit' status placed the newly founded educational institution among the so-called philanthropic institutions, which, under this designation, was partially exempt from national taxation. This exemption was justified by the development of a medical course which, as part of its function, would also provide health care for the city's population. In 1936, with this purpose in mind, the Civil Association would establish its teaching hospital, the São Paulo Hospital (SPH), whose first wards would begin to receive patients into provisional premises in 1936, and into its own facilities in 1940.

From the beginning, funding for the new hospital[39] was based on resources obtained by the School of Medicine from a range of different sources, including: (a) monthly fees paid by students; (b) quotas paid by its founders; (c) agreements entered into with federal, state and municipal governments, which released funds in the form of subventions; (d) agreements executed with the municipality and the state to finance the hospital's wards, its emergency department and hospital beds for indigents; and (e) agreements signed with pension funds and institutes, as of 1940. These pension institutes had been in development since the 1920s. In the 1930s, stimulated by the

Getúlio Vargas administration and linked to the Ministry of Labour, they expanded their coverage and activities.

The transformations that occurred in the Brazilian economy between the 1930s and 1960s attest to an intense urbanisation process that would bring with it a considerable increase in demand for social and hospital assistance. The development of Brazilian social security entailed the provision of medical, hospital and pharmaceutical services to its beneficiaries. Pension funds and institutes hired hospital services for their members. Poor people, who worked in the informal sector, remained dependent on charitable/philanthropic institutions. São Paulo Hospital, thus, followed the tradition of the houses of mercy as a non-profit institution that sought public and private resources to finance its activities. It also sought to attract the social security institutes that were developing and, at the same time, secure the autonomy of action and choice characteristic of a private enterprise.

The 1930s and 1940s saw the reinforcement of a trend in Brazilian hospital care, in which the government purchased and funded services provided by private hospitals, especially the non-profit ones. It was assumed that charitable/philanthropic institutions providing care for the poor and indigents could charge for services offered to public bodies, mainly through subventions and agreements. In the case of the SPH, whose clientele was for the most part composed of indigents, the reliance on public funding would only increase throughout the twentieth century.

The 1940s and 1950s coincided with the development of the so-called *modelo hospitalocêntrico*. This model arose from an increased demand for health care, especially in big urban centres, and from the influence of new technologies, which resulted in more expensive medical services. The hospital became, therefore, the privileged locus of these services, as it concentrated various medical specialties and provided them with the most modern and expensive equipment and infrastructure. In this context, the SPH found a way to finance its creation and the construction of its infrastructure, but not always to support its teaching activities and services.

The financial hardships faced by the School of Medicine in the 1950s, especially in maintaining teaching beds intended for indigent patients, led its members to adopt a radical solution: in 1956, the SPSM was turned into a federal institution. The SPH, though, remained a private and philanthropic institution.[40] The law that federalised the School did not include the hospital and its enormous liabilities. It made clear, however, that the hospital should offer beds for teaching activities.[41] In this way, the SPSM, now an educational institution of the public federal system, would continue to use beds in São Paulo Hospital to teach medical specialties. The hospital, in turn, would preserve the main characteristics of the original civil association, changing only its name to São Paulo Society for the Development of Medicine (SPDM), from then on considered the sponsor of the hospital. The political intentions behind this change are quite explicit in the minutes of the members' meetings of the original association. It was hoped that the federal school could obtain larger funds to finance teaching beds allocated to indigent patients and that physicians would maintain their autonomy in the management of the private hospital. It should be noted that the members of the SPH/SPDM were the same professors who came to compose the School Governing Council. This was a new articulation of the public-private mix that had been present in the SPSM's history since its inception.

Analysis of the financial statements of the original civil association, including those produced by the new Society, suggests that the professors were able to mobilise great amounts of capital for the construction of buildings, such as the Tuberculosis Dispensary. Resulting from an agreement signed with the National Tuberculosis Service and the Health Department of the Ministry of Education and Health, the dispensary was built by the National Tuberculosis Service on a piece of land owned by the School. After the dispensary's opening in

1958, the properties were divided between the School and the Society and the land passed to the ownership of the Society. Service provision would be maintained with resources from the School and also the Society, which would have to raise subventions from public authorities in order to carry out its philanthropic activities. These subventions, though, never had the necessary regularity. This can be seen as a kind of 'financial engineering' through which huge assets could be accumulated by means of agreements and loans. However, short-term expenses for the maintenance of health care services were always beset by the inconsistency of the subventions targetted at the needy.

The accounting exercise carried out by the auditor Américo Oswaldo Campiglia in 1957 at the request of the Society and the School makes patent the financing problems reported here. According to the auditor, by *'incorporating the subventions into the total revenue'*[42] as an anticipated but unrealised factor, a surplus was obtained for the period. In other words, this surplus was based on subventions yet to come, but whose regularity could never be confirmed through the accounting records. This practice therefore allowed the hospital to retain its charitable status, wtih accompanying tax privileges.

The creation of the Social Security National Institute (INPS, in the Portuguese acronym) in 1966, which replaced the old pension institutes and concentrated benefits into a single state-managed social security system, would change the role played by subventions from and agreements with the municipality and the State in the SPH/SPDM's financing. In the course of the 1970s, the importance of revenue received from the INPS in the hospital's total revenue increased significantly. A social security system was, therefore, created based on health care provided to the individual, for curative purposes and delivered in a hospital. In this system, philanthropic enterprises had great importance: they were responsible for hospitals all across Brazil and signed agreements with the INPS to provide medical assistance as established in the new model.

This type of 'articulation between public and private' characterised the development of health care in Brazil and promoted 'hybrid forms' of organising these services.[43] The experience at the complex SPH-SPDM/SPSM undoubtedly typified and consolidated the historical trajectory of public health in Brazil insofar as its existence was defined by the shared management of a private philanthropic hospital and a federal medical school.

Thus, the growth of health care funded by social security contributions from workers, employers, and the federal government became popular. Investment by the state in public health and preventive medicine was always proportionally smaller in the 1970s. The political choices that were made and put into effect, and that were evidenced by the decreasing participation of the Ministry of Health in the Union's total budget certainly explain suppressed tragedies, such as the meningitis epidemic that swept the country in the early part of the 1970s. Funds for a vaccination campaign would only be released in December 1974.[44]

This system developed since the creation of the INPS was as fragile as it was large. The charges for care by a private hospital network largely composed of philanthropic institutions, such as São Paulo Hospital and SPDM, were billed by 'Unit of Service', such as a surgical procedure, an item of equipment, an appointment, or hospitalisation costs. This was difficult to control and often became a source of corruption as doctors over-billed. An additional factor was the insufficiency of the subventions granted by the different levels of government for the care of indigent patients at the same hospitals that received social security patients. Rates paid by the INPS for medical services were also low, and the transfer of resources was not free from delays and cancellations due to the reciprocal distrust between the INPS and the contracted hospital network.

The difficulties posed by the INPS's fragile financial structure to the operationalisation of the hospital were as evident as they were serious. There were problems paying medical residents, suppliers and employees; the impossibility of providing care of the expected and requisite quality; and constant attempts by the School and the Society to renegotiate contracts with the INPS and obtain subventions that were enough to cover the deficit created by their dependence on its revenue. Moreover, the urgent need to expand the hospital, incapable of serving an ever-growing number of patients who sought treatment in its wards and emergency room, led the School to request resources from the Social Development Support Fund. This fund, created by law in 1974, aimed to 'provide financial support for social programmes and projects that comply with the guidelines and priorities of the social development strategy set out in the National Development Plan.' Through the fund, it was possible to take out loans from the Caixa Econômica Federal, a government-owned savings bank, for 'publicly relevant projects in the areas of health, sanitation, education, labour, and social security.'[45] Bearing in mind that throughout the 1970s the private hospital network, either philanthropic or not, came to be responsible for serving roughly 90% of INPS-funded patients, and that hospitals became the citizens' main gateway into the health system, the government's intentions were clear. Likewise, the difficulties in organising primary care structures, after the creation in 1988 of Brazil's national health service, the *Sistema Único de Saúde* (SUS), can also be explained when one considers the history of public policies formulated in the 1960s and 1970s.

Table 2.1 illustrates the economic difficulties reported here.[46] It is based on records of current assets and liabilities (CA and CL) of the SPH, as well as on the application of the current liquidity ratio (CLR), which signifies an institution's solvency as regards its financial obligations.

Table 2.1: Assets and Liabilities of Sao Paolo Hospital. 1960-1984 (Brazilian currency)[47]

Year	Current Assets	Current Liabilities	Current Liquidity Ratio
1960	8,035,569.8	35,694,918.6	0.22
1961	1,270,151.9	60,050,926	0.02
1962	4,753,944.1	31,666,232.2	0.15
1963	Illegible		
1964	7,401,368	114,561,286	0.06
1965	19,154,265	179,792,110	0.11
1966	88,421,801	382,709,406	0.23
1967	19,547.48	992,984.6	0.02
1968	192,690.5	841,621.37	0.22
1969	289,259.26	929,701.86	0.31
1970	848,261.76	2,504,193.36	0.33
1971	550,556.97	3,172,826.97	0.17
1972	694,885.09	4,523,954.81	0.15
1973	972,196.78	6,018,866.73	0.16
1974	3,887,079.42	5,529,588.09	0.7
1975	6,922,647.91	14,147,606.37	0.49
1976	5,690,139.01	45,749,248.33	0.12
1977	28,884,092.98	63,078,766.77	0.46
1978	57,961,378.03	136,903,243.3	0.42
1979	Illegible		
1980	113,314,806.3	209,185,299.5	0.54
1981	398,832,895.2	361,253,074.7	1.1
1982	551,624,093.9	461,988,054.6	1.19
1983	1,076,610,143	2,056,564,818	0.52
1984	3,220,251,573	6,115,197,279	0.53

The table shows liquidity ratios mostly below 1, which is evidence of the institution's insolvency. Even the years of solvency (1981-1982) only occurred because of the federalisation of the SPH's employees, which balanced the ratio between revenue and contractual liabilities for two years.[48]

According to the Minutes of the School Governing Council and of the Society Members' Meeting between the 1960s and 1990s, the perception of insolvency always led to the following proposals: (a) requests for additional municipal and state funding for emergency care delivery; (b) hiring of new staff via the school, in order not to burden the Society payroll; (c) increases in the number of private hospital beds, in order to balance the finances against the expenses with teaching beds intended for indigents; and last but surely not least, (d) requests to turn the hospital into government property. These proposals, however, had never been a consensus within the community. There had always been those who wanted the SPH to remain a private philanthropic civil association, and those who asserted the impossibility for the SPH to be funded on the historical grounds on which it had been built, thus demanding its complete federalisation.

In the process of transition from the INPS/INAMPS system to the universal and comprehensive SUS, the Society faced a serious financial crisis caused by the indebtedness of the late 1980s and by the aftermath of the economic 'miracle' promoted by the military between 1964 and 1984.[49] The transition to the 1990s would witness strikes and deficits, the likes of which had never been seen in the SPH's history.[50] When the SUS was created, 95% of the SPH's activities were funded with public resources and payments proceeding from the agreement with the INPS/INAMPS. Prior forms of financial engineering would also point the way out of the crisis: expansion, the search for new agreements and new areas of activity to increase revenue. It should be noted that, between the initiation of social security, when the school and the hospital developed, and the creation of the SUS, the Society remained a private philanthropic institution, signing agreements with ministries, state and municipal secretariats, and receiving subventions to provide public health care. The health system has undoubtedly changed, but the continuance of the SPH/SPDM amid the change indicates the difficulties in consolidating the SUS as a fully public system in which private insurance was unnecessary. These difficulties will be examined below, taking into account the very process of creation of the SUS.

The Construction of the Unified Health System

It was in the years of the military dictatorship, between 1964 and 1984, that the social security health care system reached its apex and also its crisis.[51] The control and distribution of social security resources by the state proved not only inefficient but, more importantly, unable to deliver quality health care to those entitled to it. Nor could it expand health care coverage to patients not covered by social security. A national health system was necessary, with a funding model that met citizens' needs. Sanitary Reform was also necessary. This was a movement that brought together several other social movements in the late 1970s to demand universal public health care and the country's democratisation.[52] The SUS was created by the 1988 Constitution and became a legal obligation with the 1990 laws No. 8,080 and 8,142.

As a historical process, the SUS had its practical beginning in the 1970s, with social and political movements against the dictatorship and in favour of the democratic freedoms and the democratisation of the State. These movements were expanding and intensifying their fight for a just and solidary society, and for a State with universal public policies on basic human rights. In health, these libertarian movements were strengthened by the Sanitary Reform, anticipating what would become, years later, the constitutional directives of universality, equality and community participation.[53]

As a result of the Sanitary Reform movement and the defeat of the military dictatorship in 1984, the new Constitution, promulgated in 1988 and known as the Citizen Constitution, stated:

Article 198. Public health activities and services are integrated in a regional and hierarchical network and constitute a single system, organised according to the following directives:
I – decentralisation, with a single management in each sphere of government;
II – comprehensive service, priority being given to preventive activities, without prejudice to assistance services;
III – participation of the community.
Paragraph 1. The unified health system shall be financed, as set forth in article 195, with funds from the social welfare budget of the Union, the states, the Federal District and the municipalities, as well as from other sources. (...)
Article 199. Health assistance is open to private enterprise.
Paragraph 1. Private institutions may participate in a supplementary manner in the unified health system, in accordance with the directives established by the latter, by means of public law contracts or agreements, preference being given to philanthropic and non-profit entities.[54]

This research is concerned particularly with the effects of Article 199 in relation to the principles laid down in Article 198 of the Constitution. In order to offer a full health service with the participation of the community in the making of choices and decisions, the regionalised, hierarchical and decentralised network must provide three levels of service: primary health care, which is the gateway to the SUS; medium-complexity care; and high-complexity care. Primary care is evidently provided in higher numbers and is allocated a proportionally greater amount of resources. The thirty years of existence of SUS have undoubtedly seen a substantial increase in the number of primary care service providers. This has made it possible to include a large proportion of the population in the registers of the Basic Health Units (BHU), as well as to connect BHUs with nearby medium- and high-complexity service providers. The urgency in constructing SUS, however, entailed the execution of agreements and contracts with private hospitals, as suggested in Article 199. The Society would integrate with the hospital network serving SUS patients. The same would happen with hospitals of the brotherhoods of mercy and with all other *filantrópicos* in the country. There were differences here, though, that need to be pointed out.

Among Brazilian philanthropic hospitals today, including those belonging to houses of mercy, some are characterised as general hospitals and offer services that range from outpatient care to highly-complex care. In these hospitals, some admit any type of patient in their emergency departments, whereas others are exclusively dedicated to one specialty (orthopedics, pediatrics etc.) and only receive patients for that specific specialty. Hardly any philanthropic hospital or house of mercy receives only SUS patients; most also have beds reserved for privately insured patients. In this aspect, though, hospitals differ immensely from one another. Some, like the SPH, allocate few beds for private patients. Others seek to provide services equally to SUS and private patients in an attempt to balance their finances, since payments from the SUS are allegedly insufficient. Still others, in order to secure the number of SUS beds required by law for their certification as *filantrópicos*, operate as social organisations (SO), managing public service providers. These may be either BHUs or hospitals, located or not in their vicinities. In their financial statements, these SOs record inpatient and outpatient services offered by the public service providers they manage, as if provided by themselves as their mandatory share of public services. Public patients, however, rarely make use of the private hospital's services.

At present, it is a fact that SUS is harmed by policies of underfunding, but it is also a fact that this situation affects primary care service providers more seriously than general and special hospitals. Having in mind that private health insurance plans pay more, it is easily understandable why medical corporations on hospital management boards want the expansion of private plans, leaving the SUS only for people considered extremely poor. It is important to reaffirm that, when one speaks of certification as a charitable and philanthropic entity, the legal possibility of a tax waiver by the government is involved. In other words, the legislation grants exemption from certain taxes in exchange for public services, provided for the needy population and funded by the SUS. The tax waiver necessarily entails the provision of these services, and it is in this aspect that medical corporations have great relevance. In their political actions, these corporations associate the demand for a tax waiver with the argument for the expansion of private health insurance and the decrease of their obligations towards the SUS, an attitude that compromises the universalising principles stated in the Brazilian Constitution.

Researchers of the role played by philanthropy in the SUS have drawn a distinction between traditional philanthropic entities and those following an entrepreneurial model.[55] The former, true heirs to the Christian charitable practices, provide services almost exclusively to those in need and are all but fully funded by the SUS and by supplementary public funds. This is the situation in which houses of mercy find themselves, especially those in inland towns in the state of São Paulo. The others, which generally separate facilities intended for SUS patients from those for private patients, operate politically as described above. This is the case, for example, of São Paulo *Misericórdia*, which has built facilities to receive private patients exclusively. On the other hand, São Paulo Hospital has never had, in all its history, more than 5% of its revenue derived from fully private resources, even though the Minutes of the Society Members' Meetings show the need to increase the number of private beds so as to improve funding for its activities. After the creation of the INPS, in 1966, the dependence on resources from social security was very heavy, as has been pointed out. These resources, however, were distributed and managed by the state, according to the military dictatorship's intention of universalising health care through social security, although this never materialised.

Therefore, Brazilian health care would continue to be regulated by public powers, but provided through multiple types of agreement involving institutional obligations between the public and private spheres. This historically constructed trend would be further consolidated with the 1990 Managerial Reform of the State, which gave legal status to the juridical entity of the Social Organisations.[56] These were private institutions which could also benefit from its philanthropic status, and which were incentivised to apply for the management of public service providers.

In 1994, the Society started operating joint primary care programmes with municipalities and states, independently from the activities of the Hospital. This would lead to the SPDM's certification as a SO in 1998. This expansion process of the Society, which would turn it into the most important manager of public service providers in the state of São Paulo in the early twenty-first century, was based on the SPDM's relations with the School and on its management of São Paulo Hospital, since the public medical school and its teaching hospital offered academic support that justified that expansion.

Final Considerations

Throughout the twentieth century, philanthropy was defined as publicly relevant action which was not for the pursuit of profit. According to this definition, direct-management public institutions and philanthropic institutions could be considered qualified to provide public health care services funded by the INPS/INAMPS or, after 1998, directly by the SUS. This pattern of expansion of individual health care activities resulted in the growth of the private hospital network and blurred the distinction between public and private in the Brazilian health care system.

A hybrid system was, thus, historically created which is explained by the pervasiveness of *misericordia* and *filantrópicos* in Brazil and by the urgency of structuring a unified health system after 1988.[57] This situation also opened a private gateway into SUS which competes with public spaces and services, within these very hospitals, for public funding. This competition takes place in different ways, since the SPH, as discussed here, has always received patients coming mostly from the INPS/INAMPS or the SUS, whereas *Albert Einstein Hospital*, for example, despite being considered a philanthropic hospital according to the same regulations, gives preference to private patients. A single group of laws promotes distinct inequalities. This is possible because large philanthropic hospitals can be accredited as SOs and remotely manage public service providers, leaving their own beds out of the equation.

Any assumption that Brazil has transitioned from philanthropy-linked charity, which characterised its early health care experience, to public health, is refuted by the resilience of historically constructed medical practices and public service management practices. What is more, these practices have been sanctioned by the same Constitution that stated the universality of the right to health. In this context, the connection between private charity/philanthropy and public funding explained private charity's difficulty in collecting enough donations. At the same time, the government considered that building hospitals and organising health care for the entire population with physicians, assistants and nurses directly paid by the Treasury was too steep an investment.

The Christian and private origins of charitable and/or philanthropic practices impacted the contemporary construction of citizenship, given that Brazilian hospital provision has always been located between citizenship entitlement and hierarchical benevolence, between the possibilities of creation of public spaces and the permanence of private actions that establish themselves as public, thus taking the place of the state. These private activities receive tax exemption privileges and select their clientele and their areas of operation without regard to the public interest. Moreover, Christian compassion, the basis for charitable actions, brought with itself a hierarchy between charitable givers and receivers. These latter never participated in the political decisions concerning how to relieve suffering caused by poverty and disease. Most of the time, it was nothing but charitable compassion enfolded into social hierarchies that were thus legitimised.[58]

If solidarity was at the basis of what some Enlightenment thinkers proposed for a world based on the pact among equal citizens, the survival of Christian charity in the health care structures developed in Brazil since the nineteenth century has hampered the understanding of health care as a universal right. The idea of Christian private charity had a public dimension and became, in the Brazilian experience, a political motivation for segmentation of clientele and for obtaining private advantages. This, however, is history under construction. The SUS, Brazil's greatest social achievement after the end of the military dictatorship, belongs to all Brazilians, who are still awaiting its effective consolidation.

1. This research is funded by Fundação do Amparo à Pesquisa do Estado de SãoPaulo (FAPESP), Process 2017 / 16721-0

2. For an overview of recents research, see Isabel dos Guimarães Sá, Quando o rico se faz pobre: Misericórdias, caridade e poder no Império português (1500-1800) (Lisbon: CNCDP, 1997); Idem As misericórdias portuguesas – séculos XVI a XVIII (R. J.: FGV, 2013); Laurinda Abreu, The political and social dynamics of poverty, poor relief and health care in early-modern Portugal (N. Y.: Routledge, 2016).

3. Renato Franco, Pobreza e caridade leiga – as Santas Casas de Misericórdia na América Portuguesa (PhD thesis, School of Philosophy, Languages and Human Sciences, University of São Paulo, São Paulo, 2011).

4. Sá, op. cit. (note 2).

5. Sá, op. cit. (note 2); Charles Boxer, O Império marítimo português (1415-1825). (Lisbon: Edições 70, 2011).

6. Boxer, ibid.; A. J. R. Russell-Wood, Fidalgos e filantropos – A Santa Casa de Misericórdia da Bahia, 1550-1755 (Brasília: Editora da UnB, 1981). It is important to highlight the relevance of Russell-Wood's work for the understanding of the misericórdias in the Portuguese Empire. In the case of São Paulo, however, even if one considers the structuring role of mercies in the Portuguese Empire, the poverty of the village suggests cautions in the analysis. When São Paulo began its economic expansion at the beginning of the nineteenth century, we were already experiencing the winds of independence. And that is why the misericódia of the village of São Paulo connected the contents of Christian charity with the new political guidelines of the free Province, also led by an elite that changed itself, appropriating the experience of the misericórdia.

7. R.T.Santos, 'Social Innovation Oriented towards Solving Pratical Problems. The Case of the Santa Casa da Misericórdia de Lisboa', in C.Ruiz, Viñals and C. Parra Rodríguez (eds), Social Innovation: New Forms of Organisation in Knowledge-Based Societies (Abingdon: Routledge, 2015), 84-108, at 95-6.

8. Maria Antónia Lopes and José Pedro Paiva, 'Introdução',Portugaliae Monumenta Misericordiarum – Sob o signo da mudança: de D. José I a 1834 (Lisbon: União das Misericórdias portuguesas, 2002, Vol. 7).

9. Lopes and Paiva, ibid., 31.

10. Frances Fox Piven and Richard Cloward, Regulating the poor: the functions of public welfare (N. Y.: Vintage Books, 1993).

11. Isabel dos Guimarães Sá and Maria Antónia Lopes, História Breve das Misericórdias Portuguesas, 1498-2000 (Coimbra: Imprensa da Universidade, 2008); Maria Antónia Lopes 'A intervenção da Coroa nas instituições de protecção social de 1750 a 1820', Revista de história das Ideias, 29 (2008), 131-176.

12. Russell-Wood, op. cit. (note 4).

13. For an overview of important research about the Brotherhood of the São Paulo Holy House of Mercy, see Laima Mesgravis A Santa casa de Misericórdia de São Paulo (1599?-1884) – Contribuição ao estudo da

assistência social no Brasil (S. P.: Conselho Estadual de Cultura, 1977); Glauco Carneiro O poder da Misericórdia – A Santa Casa de São Paulo (S. P.: Press, 1986). For an overview of recent research about São Paulo in this period, see Rafael Mantovani Modernizar a ordem em nome da saúde: a São Paulo de militares, pobres e escravos (1805-1840) (R. J.: Fiocruz, 2017).

14. Mesgravis, ibid.

15. Mesgravis, ibid.

16. Maria Antónia Lopes, 'A intervenção da Coroa nas instituições de protecção social de 1750 a 1820', Revista de história das Ideias, 29 (2008), 131-176.

17. Maria Antónia Lopes, ibid.

18. Foundling wheels were mechanisms embedded in an aperture in the wall of an institution whose purpose was to receive abandoned infants. They were usually found in brotherhoods of mercy which cared for the children. Child-rearing costs were usually shared between the houses of mercy and city councils.

19. Lopes and Paiva, op. cit. (note 6); Isabel dos Guimarães Sá and Maria Antónia Lopes ibid.
Laurinda Abreu has stressed the similarities between Portuguese and English legislation against vagrancy during the sixteenth and seventeenth centuries. This is an important historiographical debate that will not be considered here, where the focus is on the Christian aspects of the Luso-Brazilian experience of the mercies and their inflections during the Enlightenment era. See Abreu, Laurinda, *ibid.*

20. During the Brazilian colonial period, the sertanistas were men who ventured into the sertões (lands of the hinterland of the colony) in search of richness and indigenous populations to imprison. In São Paulo, the sertanistas were called 'bandeirantes'. Tropeiro is the designation given to Paulistas who, from the seventeenth century onwards set up commissions, or caravans, to trade horses, mules, and other products of daily use.

21. Sérgio Buarque de Holanda, Caminhos e fronteiras (S. P.: Cia das Letras, 1994).

22. Luiz Antônio de Souza Botelho e Mourão, known as the Majorat of Mateus, ruled the São Paulo Captaincy between 1765 and 1775. Ana Paula Médicci 'De capitania a província: o lugar de São Paulo nos projetos de Império, 1782-1822', in: Wilma Peres Costa and Cecília Helena de Salles Oliveira (eds), De um Império a outro – Formação do Brasil, séculos XVIII e XIX, (São Paulo: Hucitec/Fapesp, 2007); Alcir Lenharo, As tropas da moderação (São Paulo: Símbolo, 1979); Maria Odila Leite da Silva Dias A interiorização da metrópole e outros estudos (São Paulo: Alameda, 2005)

23. Franco, op. cit. (note 2); Luciana Gandelman Mulheres para um Império: órfãs e caridade nos recolhimentos femininos da Santa Casa de Misericórdia—Salvador, Rio de Janeiro e Porto – século XVIII (Campinas: Unicamp, 2005, PhD thesis); Tânia S. Pimenta 'Hospital da Santa Casa de Misericórdia: assistência à saúde no Rio de Janeiro dos Oitocentos',Anais do XXVI Simpósio Nacional de História – ANPUH (S. P., July 2011. Available on: http://www.snh2011.anpuh. org/resources/anais/14/1300881656_AR-

QUIVO_TaniaPimentatexto.pdf Accessed in February 2015).

24. Márcia Regina Barros da Silva, 'Santa Casa de Misericórdia de São Paulo: saúde e assistência se tornam públicas (1875-1910)', Varia História, 26 (44) (2010), 395-420; Idem 'Concepção de saúde e doença nos debates parlamentares paulistas entre 1830 e 1900', in: Maria L. Mott and Gisele Sanglard (eds.), História da saúde em São Paulo: instituições e patrimônio arquitetônico (1808-1958) (Barueri, SP: Minha Editora, 2011), 63-92.

25. Mantovani, op. cit. (note 10).

26. Laima Mesgravis, ibid; Wilma Peres Costa and Cecília helana de Salles Oliveira, ibid.

27. Silva, op. cit. (note 17).

28. Ibid., 70. (Author's translation)

29. There is a huge body of different studies on the First Brazilian Republic philanthropy that points out its patterns. I highlight just a few: André Mota Tropeços da medicina Bandeirante – Medicina paulista entre 1892-1920 (São Paulo: Edusp,2003); Gisele Sanglard Entre os salões e o laboratório – Guilherme Guinle, a saúde e a ciência no Rio de Janeiro, 1920-1940 (R. J.: Fiocruz, 2008); Cláudia Maria Ribeiro Viscardi 'Pobreza e assistência no Rio de Janeiro na Primeira República', História, Ciências, Saúde – Manguinhos, 18 (2011), 179-197.

30. Donna T. Andrew, Philanthropy and police (Princeton: Princeton University Press, 1989); Andrew Wear (ed.), Medicine in society (New York: Cambridge University Press, 1998).

31. David Rosner, A once charitable enterprise (Cambridge: Cambridge University Press, 2004); David J. Rothman, The Discovery of the asylum (Boston: Little Brown, 1971); American charities (N. Y.: Thomas Y Crowell Company Publishers, 1894).

32. ANTT, Hospital de São José, Livro 0947; Lopes and Paiva, op. cit. (note 6); Sá and Lopes, op. cit. (note 13); Maria Antónia Lopes, 'Os pobres e a assistência pública', in: Luis Reis Torgal and João L. Roque, História de Portugal – O liberalismo (Lisbon: Editorial Estampa, 1998), 427-437.

33. Gisele Sanglard, ibid.

34. Maria Lúcia Moot, Henrique S. Francisco, Olga Sofia F. Alves, Karla Maestrini and Douglas C. Afonso da Silva 'Assistência à saúde, filantropia e gênero: as sociedades civis na cidade de São Paulo (1893-1929)', in: Maria L. Mott and Gisele Sanglard (eds.), História da saúde em São Paulo: instituições e patrimônio arquitetônico (1808-1958) (Barueri, SP: Minha Editora, 2011), 93-132.

35. Ana Nemi (ed), EPM/SPDM – Histórias de gente, ensino e atendimento à saúde (São Paulo: Editora Fap/Unifesp, 2012); Ana Nemi Entre o público e o privado: Hospital São Paulo e Escola Paulista de Medicina (1933 a 1988) (São Paulo: Hucitec, 2020).

36. Silva, op. cit. (note 17); Mesgravis, op. cit. (note 10).

37. Maria Alice Rosa Ribeiro, História sem fim ... Inventário da saúde pública (São Paulo: Ed. da Unesp, 1993); Rodolfo Telarolli Jr. Poder e saúde – As epidemias e a formação dos serviços de saúde em São Paulo (S. P.:

Editora da Unesp, 1996); Gilberto Hochman A era do saneamento (São Paulo: HUCITEC, 2006).

38. Ana Nemi and Ewerton L. F. M. Silva, 'Imigração portuguesa e psiquiatria na capital paulista dos anos 30: modernidade e nacionalismo no atendimento à saúde', in: André Mota and Gabriela Marinho (eds.), Saúde e História de Migrantes e Imigrantes. Direitos, Instituições e Circularidades (São Paulo: FMUSP, UFABC & Casa de Soluções Editora, 2014), 43-58.

39. In order to understand the origin of the resources used by the SPH, its Accounting Books and Financial Statements have been analysed, as well as the Annals of the São Paulo municipal and state assemblies, and of the National Congress.

40. Ana Nemi, 'A federalização da Escola Paulista de Medicina: imbricações de origem entre a norma e a experiência (1956-1970)', Tempo Brasileiro, v. 178 (2009), 165-213.

41. Act No. 2,712 of 21 January 1956. Available on: http://legis.senado.leg.br/sicon/#/pesquisa/lista/documentos Accessed in April 2019. According to article 2 of the law: *'For the teaching of the São Paulo School of Medicine's specialties, the São Paulo Hospital's sponsor will ensure, through a clause in the deed referred to in this article, the use of its general wards, facilities and equipment, regardless of any payment.'*

42. Governing Council Minutes, Book VI, Minute No. 100 (02 August 1957), 46. UNIFESP President's Office Archive. An explanation was requested from the auditor about the SPSM's and the SPH's balance sheets regarding the years before and after the federalisation, in addition to a study of their respective properties after part of the SPSM's assets were incorporated into the Union.

43. Telma M. G. Menicucci Público e privado na política de Assistência à saúde no Brasil: atores, processos e trajetória (Rio de Janeiro: Fiocruz, 2007), 34 and 46.

44. Gastão W. S. Campos, Emerson E. Merhy and Everardo D. Nunes, Planejamento sem normas (São Paulo: HUCITEC, 1989); José Carlos de Souza Braga and Sérgio Goes Paula, Saúde e previdência: estudos de política social (São Paulo: CEBES/HUCITEC, 1981).

45. Law No. 6,168 of 9 December 1974. Federal Senate's Archive. Available on: http://legis.senado.leg.br/sicon/#/pesquisa/lista/documentos. Accessed in April 2019.

46. The table was constructed from the reading of: a. São Paulo Hospital's Accounting Books, Books 1565-1606, b. Minutes of the São Paulo Society for the Development of Medicine's Annual Meeting, 1960-2015. SPDM Archive.

47. From 1960 to 1984 Brazil had two different currencies: cruzeiro (1964-1967 and 1970-1984) and cruzeiro novo (1967-1970).

48. The SPSM, as a federal public school, negotiated with the Ministry of Education and Culture (MEC) the inclusion of part of the SPH's employees on the Union's payroll. The aim was to cut costs with SPH/SPDM personnel and improve the quality of the teaching at the hospital beds available for this purpose.

49. In 1977, the dictatorial military government divided the INPS into two institutions: the National Social Security Medical Assistance Institute (INAMPS, in the Portuguese acronym), an agency responsible for public health services, and the Social Security Financial Administration Institute (IAPAS, in the Portuguese acronym), responsible for finance management. In this study, we opted for using the combined acronym INPS/INAMPS to make the continuity clear.

50. 'Strike impacts school and hospital in São Paulo', in: Folha de São Paulo, 14 August 1991; 'Health crisis: ER closure causes chain reaction', in: Jornal da Tarde, 24 December 1991.

51. Braga and Paula, op. cit.(note 34).

52. Sarah Escorel, Reviravolta na Saúde: origem e articulação do movimento sanitário (Rio de Janeiro: FIOCRUZ, 1999); Jairnilson Paim O que é o SUS (Rio de Janeiro: Fiocruz, 2009).

53. Nelson Rodrigues dos Santos, 'SUS, política pública de Estado: seu desenvolvimento instituído e instituinte e a busca de saídas', Ciênc. saúde coletiva [online], vol.18, n.1, (2013) 274. (Author's translation)

54. Constituição da República federativa do Brasil (1988). (Brasília: 2008). (Author's translation)

55. Ministério da Saúde, Rede hospitalar filantrópica no Brasil: perfil histórico-institucional e ofertas de serviços (Belo Horizonte, 2001); Instituto de Pesquisa Econômica Aplicada. Financiamento Público da saúde: uma história a procura de rumo (Rio de Janeiro, 2013); idem, Radiografia do gasto tributário em saúde – 2003-2013 (Brasília, 2016).

56. Ministério da Administração Federal e Reforma do Estado, A Reforma do Estado dos anos 90: Lógica e mecanismos de controle (Brasília: 1997); Ana Nemi and Lilia B. Schraiber, 'Luiz Carlos Bresser-Pereira: o Sistema Único de Saúde (SUS) e a Reforma Gerencial do Estado dos anos de 1990', Interface (Botucatu. Online), v. 23 (2019), 1-13.

57. Margareth C. Portela, Sheyla M. L. Lima, Pedro R. Barbosa, Miguel M. Vasconcelos, Maria Alícia D. Ugá and Silvia Gerschman, 'Caracterização assistencial de hospitais filantrópicos no Brasil', Revista de saúde pública, 2004; 38 (6): 811-8.

58. Hannah Arendt, A condição humana (R. J.: Forense Universitária, 1993); idem, Sobre a revolução (S. P.: Companhia das Letras, 2011).

Chapter 3

Principles and Problems of Hospital Funding in Germany in the Twentieth Century

Axel C. Hüntelmann
(Charité—University Medicine Berlin)

Nearly every historical or contemporary publication dealing with health insurance and hospital economics in West Germany since the 1960s starts by complaining about the deficiencies of the current health care system and its lack of funding.[1] Be the authors hospital physicians, complaining about their out-dated or missing equipment, or politicians, railing against the rising costs of hospitals and medical technology, regardless of the money spent, it is never enough.

Since the late 1960s, numerous expert commissions, established by the government, have analysed and proposed reforms to the West German health care system and hospital funding. The result has been a near-perpetual reign of reform: no sooner has one structural reform been elaborated and implemented, than a new initiative gets underway designed to reduce health care costs, especially hospital expenditures.[2] As to the causes of the rise in health care expenditure, government officials and health care policy experts have identified ever more expensive technical equipment, an overcapacity of beds, and a general lack of efficient cost management. Hospital economists have suggested reducing bed capacities and improving hospital management, while financial experts recommend competition between hospitals and health care institutions as a means of reducing costs. Such policy prescriptions have prompted German politicians, health care professionals, and patient groups to complain about an increasing economisation and commodification of health care.[3]

Although at a first glance the debate about the economisation of health care and insufficient hospital funding seems to be relatively new, in fact it dates back at least to the late eighteenth or early nineteenth century when the hospital became a "modern" medical institution.[4] But in contrast to the large number of political publications complaining about insufficient resources and suggesting improvements to hospital finance, there have been only a few publications addressing the history of hospital finance in Germany. Whereas for Britain there exists a rich literature on the history of hospital accounting[5] and finance,[6] for Germany there are only few local case studies, mainly focussed on the early modern period and the nineteenth century.[7]

Sometimes publications dealing with current hospital management issues sketch the history of hospital finance, but mainly as a pre-history to more contemporary developments or problems in the second half of the twentieth century.[8] And these publications pay scant attention to the socio-political and cultural historical background. Publications on the history of public health care in twentieth century Germany likewise ignore or marginalise hospital finance. The same is true for historical studies on medical institutions, which have focused first and foremost on hospitals and medical faculties during the national socialist era or—inspired by the work of Michel Foucault and because of rich source material—on the history of mental hospitals.

In light of these historiographic shortcomings, this text examines the principles and development of hospital funding and finance in Germany in the twentieth century and major shifts in this history. An analysis of hospital funding can facilitate broader insight into the structure and financing of public health care in Germany. It also illuminates the interrelationship between health insurance and hospital funding, and the effects and problems it has spawned. As a consequence of the shift from care to cure, as hospitals were transformed into medical institutions in the nineteenth century, hospital expenses increased (as did national health care budgets). As part of this process, hospitals were forced to reduce costs at any price and, as I argue, in the last decades of the twentieth century the hospital's character changed from a charitable or welfare institution and a public enterprise, which served and was responsible to the community, into a profit-orientated enterprise. This transformation has led to ongoing conflicts between neo-liberal ideas and profit-driven goals on the one hand, and humanistic ideals and practical health care concerns on the other; conflicts between neo-liberal and social health care policy experts, between hospital managers, physicians and hospital staff. As both social welfare institutions and as important components of public health care systems, hospitals have for more than a century been hailed as features of modernity and progress, essential to the preservation of the healthy fighting and working bodies needed to defend the country (in the inter-national struggle for survival) and to enhance the national stock of human capital. But over the past few decades, with the rapid economisation of medicine and commodification of health care, health has been reduced to a cost-factor in debates about ailing public finances.

In addressing the principles and prehistory of hospital funding in Germany in the nineteenth and early twentieth century, this text relies on secondary literature on the history of hospitals, hospital finances, and public health care. For the second half of the twentieth century, the study is based on contemporary sources and manuals about hospital economics and management.

I will begin with a sketch of the German system of hospital finance, starting with principles that had evolved in the early modern period and during the nineteenth century. Then I describe the establishment of statutory health insurance in the 1880s and its importance for hospital funding, followed by sections on changes during the Wilhelmine Empire, the Weimar Republic, and the 1930s. I then summarise the history of hospital finance in the 1950s and 1960s, before a longer section describes developments since the 1970s during a period of ongoing reforms. Due to limitations of space, these sections focus mainly on West Germany. I conclude by analysing the changes and problems of hospital funding in Germany during the twentieth century.

Pre-history of hospital finance in Germany until the introduction of statutory health insurance

The history of hospital finance in Germany (and especially the health insurance laws of the 1880s) is incomprehensible without taking account of its prehistory. In the middle ages and in early modern times, hospitals were commonly hospices, alms houses and infirmaries. At this time there was little difference between hospitals in German territories and other states.[9] This changed during an era of absolutist state-building and the establishment of statehood in competing German principalities. In absolutist states, population policy and public health care were issues of public order and the common good was deemed to be the responsibility of the state or sovereign, as articulated in publications on population policy by Johann Peter Süßmilch or on medical police by Johann Peter Frank.[10]

Up until the end of the nineteenth century, hospital operating costs were comprised mainly of expenses for staff, food, clothing, lighting, heating, and the maintenance of buildings and furniture. Medical treatment and instruments comprised only a small fraction of a hospital's outlay.[11] The structure of hospital expenses changed after 1900, a development that also prompted efforts to increase hospital income, as we will see below.

In the early nineteenth century, hospitals were owned mostly by cities, the state or the church. The owners of large hospitals usually provided the land, buildings and various forms of funding. Having often originated from earlier donations of land or capital, hospitals generated income from capital interest or rents of land and houses, such as Hubertus-Spital in Düsseldorf or Julius-Spital in Würzburg,[12] or from contributions made by prosperous landed estates. Furthermore, some hospitals generated income from privileges granted to them by the state (like special customs, taxes or fees for certificates),[13] from cultivating land, or from profit yielded by the hospital's own household economy. Another important source of income was government or municipal subsidies granted especially for treating the poor. Hospital owners would normally reimburse hospitals for budget overruns.[14] University hospitals and medical schools were special cases: their educational responsibilities imposed additional costs which, in turn, had to be subsidised by the state. During the nineteenth century, as a proportion of hospital income, donations decreased rapidly, while at the same time state and municipal subsidies grew.[15]

By 1800, hospitals in Germany were already generating revenue from patient fees and this source of income increased rapidly during the nineteenth century.[16] Dating back to early modern times, guilds had 'rented' their 'own' rooms in hospices where members (especially journeymen) were cared for when sick or injured; and over time these arrangements evolved into hospital subscription schemes. Furthermore, since the early nineteenth century various forms of voluntary health and hospital insurance plans helped establish and fund hospitals.[17] In Bremen and Würzburg, for instance, associations of craftsmen and domestic servants were established to pay for members' hospital care or treatment.[18] From the 1830s, population growth, urbanisation, and the erosion of traditional communities prompted municipalities to establish guild- and employer-based insurance schemes. As a result, from mid-century various forms of (sometimes mandatory) local health insurance or hospital subscription plans became a permanent source of hospital revenue. In the long run, it appears that the establishment of statutory health insurance in the German Empire in 1883 was part of a structural shift rather than a turning point or milestone in the history of the welfare state.[19]

Establishment of statutory health insurance in Germany and its consequences for hospital funding

In June 1883, the German government began implementing a statutory health insurance programme for industrial workers with an annual income less than 2,000 marks, soon to be followed by accident insurance in 1884, and old age pension insurance in 1889. Both workers and their employers contributed to the health insurance programme, which was based on principles of reciprocity and solidarity, meaning that every person paying contributions was entitled to certain benefits: visits to the doctor, medication, hospital care, and limited sick-pay were covered. *Prima facie*, the programme aimed to protect industrial workers in case of temporary illness and prevent them from becoming impoverished. In principle, however, the health insurance programmes merely centralised the existing system of municipal and regional health insurance schemes. Furthermore, health insurance was not the main focus of Bismarck's social security legislation and was designed only to bridge the period following an accident and to cover claims related to industrial injuries. For this reason, the benefits were limited to the insured worker and did not extend to other family members. Furthermore, in the mid-1880s only about ten per cent of the population was included in the programme. And finally, the government established social insurance with the aim of pacifying and co-opting the working class after having implemented anti-Socialist legislation in 1878 that outlawed the Social Democrat Party and suppressed workers' rights to organise.[20]

In subsequent decades, statutory health insurance had—albeit often limited—consequences for hospitals and hospital funding because more people had access to and were able to afford hospital treatment. In addition, the number of people willing to visit hospitals was increasing, mainly for two reasons. First and foremost, with improvements in medical therapy more people placed their hopes in hospital treatment, resulting in a rise in the number of in-patient admissions. Second, older health funds had different payment schemes: most resolved claims by disbursing money directly to the member as compensation for lost income (or medical treatment); others executed payments for medical services directly to physicians or hospitals. In the first case, members often preferred to take the money, purchase medication, and remain home in order to avoid expensive hospital visits. After the introduction of statutory health insurance, members were compensated for income loss *and* had access to hospital care.[21]

After statutory health insurance had been implemented, a great number of local health insurance associations were founded and registered with the Imperial Insurance Office. Some of these associations had emerged from older associations of factory workers, guilds, and occupational associations. Of varying size, ranging from hundreds to thousands of members, these groups soon amalgamated into larger district organisations.[22] In subsequent decades, more and more workers and employees became members of health insurance funds, which in turn generated additional burdens on hospitals' administrative staff.

In general, a hospital charged patients for the number of days they had stayed at the hospital, based on a daily rate that covered hospital operating costs, like food and accommodation. At the end of a patient's hospital stay, in addition to the daily rates, hospitals also billed for more expensive medical treatments.[23] Billing procedures varied depending on the patient's status: if patients stayed at the hospital of their own account, they were billed directly and had to pay part of their bill in advance. If patients were insured or impoverished, they had to provide evidence of their membership of an insurance programme or present official certification of their indigence in order to ensure that their hospital expenses would be paid for by the municipal welfare authority. Costly medical treatment often had to be pre-approved by health insurance or welfare officials if they were to reimburse hospitals for the additional expenses.[24]

Changes in hospital funding around 1910

Between the 1880s and the 1910s, German society witnessed a demographic and sociopolitical sea change: the population grew rapidly from 41 million in 1871 to 64 million people by 1910, and people from the countryside migrated into overcrowded cities. Besides urbanisation, rapid industrialisation compromised the working and living conditions of large parts of the population. The German Empire became a leading industrial nation, entangled in numerous international conflicts in the era of imperialism. On the other hand, mortality rates declined as food production improved, infectious diseases were checked, new medical innovations were introduced, and new hospitals and other medical institutions were constructed. The health of the nation's population manifested itself in falling rates of mortality and morbidity; rising numbers of hospital beds were considered to be signs of progress and modernity.[25] In Berlin, for instance, where the population more than doubled from 826,000 in 1871 to 1.9 million in 1900, the Charité hospital was complemented by four new community hospitals, founded between 1872 and 1906. The growing number of physicians trained at medical schools facilitated medical innovations and specialisation; in addition to municipal and confessional hospitals, numerous small private clinics were established, usually owned and operated by consultants, housed in regular apartments or houses, and often counting only a small number of beds.[26]

These developments not only increased the number of patients but changed their status as well. In 1883, only a small proportion of the national population had been eligible to benefit from statutory health insurance, but by 1914 nearly all sectors of production, trade and agriculture were included. In addition to workers, servants and craftsmen, salaried employees as well as their relatives could now also receive benefits.[27] Consolidated in district organisations, health insurance funds expanded their bargaining power vis-à-vis general practitioners. This led to a number of serious disputes between health insurance funds and physicians, to doctors' strikes, and to the foundation of the "Hartmannbund", a professional association aiming 'to protect the economic interests of physicians and the medical profession'.[28] By comparison, health insurance funds had little leverage when it came to bargaining with municipal and state hospitals which treated hundreds and thousands of patients. Funds offset this imbalance by diversifying the health care benefits they offered to their members.

As they incorporated new medical innovations and expensive therapies, hospitals modified their accounting practices and scheduled special tariffs for novel treatments like chemo- or serum therapy and for laboratory analyses and other diagnostic techniques like x-rays. After 1900 hospitals started to publish leaflets showing their daily rates, dietary schemes and charges for medical services.[29] What started, for instance, at the community hospital in Düsseldorf around 1910 as a four-page leaflet soon became a twelve-page brochure in the 1920s.[30] As a consequence of these innovations, costs per patient rose from 11.05 marks in 1885 to 28.49 marks in 1914,[31] which spawned renewed complaints about rising costs for medical care and hospital treatment.[32] But beyond treatment usually covered by health insurance, special services were listed for different classes of patients. For example, the brochure of the Düsseldorf community hospital listed additional services for first-class patients like special meals or larger hospital rooms.[33] The differentiation helped to attract middle- and upper-class patients who might previously have avoided hospitals which were still struggling to overcome their reputation as working-class or pauper institutions. By offering more expensive services and accommodation, hospitals could generate additional income directly from the patient. These additional services point to a characteristic of the German system that is valid to this day: hospitals charge standard rates for medical services covered by statutory health insurance, but alternatively, if patients are enrolled in private health insurance plans (or willing to pay additional expenses on their own), they can receive extra services.

Another characteristic of German health insurance funds was their autonomous self-administration, with employees and employers equally represented in their supervising committees.[34] Employee representatives tried to expand—often successfully—the range of medical services covered by their plans,[35] helping to attract new members in competition with other funds.[36] A steady influx of new, healthy employees allowed funds to provide more generous benefits. But for smaller funds, a few cases of severe illness could put their solvency at risk. It turned out that many smaller funds had overextended themselves, forcing them to either reduce their benefits or go bankrupt. On occasion the Imperial Insurance Office had to intervene. As a consequence of these risks, social security programs were substantially revised, and the Imperial Insurance Code enforced in 1911. The so-called *Reichsversicherungsordnung* came into force on 1 January 1914 and remained essentially unchanged until the 1970s. The new code standardised funds and services, enlarged the group of people included in statutory health insurance, diminished the influence of employees in the committees and prescribed that health insurance funds had to have a minimum number of members. All these measures were thought to consolidate the funds' financial situation and reduce the risk of bankruptcy.[37]

Changes in hospital funding in the 1920s

The First World War and post-war turmoil delayed the effects of the Imperial Insurance Code on hospitals and hospital finance until 1919. Indeed, well into the 1920s, hospitals confronted a number of severe problems which can be illustrated using the example of the Charité hospital in Berlin. During the war, many Charité physicians had been called up for military service causing a shortage of staff at a time when hospitals also had to treat wounded soldiers. In addition to the political turmoil,[38] the war's effects on public health saw hospitals struggling to cope with rising numbers of patients, especially invalided veterans and malnourished patients with deficiency diseases. Food shortages, rising prices and ultimately the hyperinflation of 1923 all placed severe strains on hospital finances.[39] Staff wages were also rising: before the war it had been common for nurses and ward staff to work ten to twelve hours a day; but at the end of the war public institutions were forced to pay standard wages and implement the eight-hour workday. Thus, hospitals had to hire additional staff to compensate for the reduced working hours.

The Charité also faced additional problems specific to its role as a military hospital, subsidised by the war ministry and responsible for educating and employing military surgeons. The demobilisation of military staff caused further personnel shortages and a reduction in subsidies, thus requiring new civilian staff to be hired and again boosting personnel costs.[40]

All of this turmoil was reflected in the hospital's accounting practices during and after the war: since 1915, no regular budget had been drafted; the budget for 1916 had simply been extended every year until 1924; and the Charité operated on quarterly financial reports used to justify ongoing state subsidies. Whereas before the war hospital administrators had meticulously calculated daily catering rates, after the war existing rates were simply adjusted for inflation.[41]

One way of dealing with rising expenditures and generating more revenue involved increasing the daily catering rates or the fees charged for medical services and treatment. But galloping inflation soon made the calculation of daily rates impractical. Furthermore, at times of hyperinflation, the pre-payment of hospital charges became problematic in the case of long-term patients. And because economic turmoil exacerbated the inability of patients and health insurance funds to pay for medical services, the hospital's outstanding accounts ballooned and often remained unsettled for longer periods of time, sometimes having to be written off entirely. To make a long story short: expenditures rose much faster than income, generating enormous deficits. Public hospital owners, who previously had subsidised these deficits, now shortened or cut public funding due to their own financial straits. To finance short-term funding gaps, hospitals like the Charité accumulated enormous liabilities which came due in the post-war period. Although the situation stabilised after the currency reform in 1924, tensions remained well into the 1920s and were revived five years later by the global economic crisis and the Great Depression.[42]

Exacerbating these difficulties, health insurance funds did not simply acquiesce to rising daily hospital rates. As a result of the Imperial Insurance Code, health insurance funds had merged and, representing thousands of insured members, had become large and powerful organisations. Faced with their own financial challenges, health insurance funds also had to cut spending drastically and began pushing general practitioners into contracts with lower fees for medical treatment or establishing so-called ambulatories (*Ambulatorien*),[43] i.e. out-patient polyclinics run and staffed by health insurance funds themselves. General practitioners and hospitals viewed these facilities as a major threat to their market dominance in the area of medical services.[44] Health insurance funds also began to question the amount and composition of daily hospital rates in the 1920s. For instance, one local health insurance fund (AOK) asked the Municipal Hospital in Düsseldorf why its daily rates were higher than those of other local and regional hospitals.[45] Rising costs and the composition of rate-schedules became an on-going topic in discussions between health insurance funds, hospitals and public health institutions.[46]

Also in the mix were a diverse array of private clinics that had evolved especially since the 1890s. Some of these facilities counted only a couple of beds and were located in apartment blocks, often in the neighbourhood of a consultant's practice. Medical school professors sometimes 'owned' these private clinics or else they rented and maintained rooms or beds in larger hospitals, where they treated wealthy patients. Often these clinics existed only for a couple of years and then vanished. These private clinics, with the notable exception of larger sanatoria, were relatively small; they filled a medical niche, and their owners were consultants or medical specialists. Furthermore, they were often exclusive, offering specialised, costly, or alternative treatments. And because they were not registered and reimbursed by health insurance schemes, conflicts between them were rare.[47]

After a short period of economic stability, discussions about cost cutting started all over again during the world economic crisis in the early 1930s. In these conflicts, funds became even more important because nearly all professional groups and their family members were covered by statutory health insurance. In addition, the introduction of unemployment insurance in the 1920s saw the unemployed also being covered by health insurance funds, as were retirees in the 1930s. At the beginning of the 1930s, payments from health insurance funds had become the main source of hospital income.[48] However, disputes about hospital financing demonstrate the plurality of actors involved in negotiations on different institutional, local, regional, and national levels: health insurance funds representing employers and employees, physicians and other medical practitioners, as well as hospitals (all of which were represented by their respective district or national associations) interacted with public health and regulatory institutions, like the Imperial Insurance Office or the Ministries of Interior or Health, with municipalities or public-private corporations (like the Red Cross or the church), or other hospital owners, and finally even with political parties of all stripes. But in subsequent years, this pluralism came to an end.

The monistic structure of hospital funding and other changes in the National Socialist era

After the National Socialist Party had come to power, it used the conflicts between hospitals, practitioners and insurance funds as an occasion to intervene in health policy and restrict the contractually-agreed rights of health insurance funds, physicians and hospitals. As concerns hospital funding,[49] these restrictions began in August 1933 when health insurance funds were prohibited from offering health care services like the above mentioned ambulatories.[50] In addition, a third-party agent was installed to mediate between and resolve conflicts of interest: the Association of Statutory Health Insurance Physicians [*Kassenärztliche Vereinigung*]. The Association negotiated fees and prices centrally and processed the settlement of bills and the distribution of payments. Only physicians who were organised in this centralised and semi-public association were allowed to bill insured patients and, vice versa, payments for insured patients were processed through the Association. *Prima facie*, the Association should pacify conflicts between health insurance funds and physicians. But the closure of out-patient facilities run by health insurance funds was designed to dismiss Jewish and socialist physicians who often held these posts. The *Kassenärztliche Vereinigung* became an obligatory and narrow clearing house for insurance payments and, because only 'Aryan' physicians could become members of the Association, Jewish (and socialist) practitioners were excluded from this vital source of income. They were only allowed to treat private Jewish patients, and, for a while, to work in privately-run clinics. The foundation of the Association has to be understood as an effort to centralise and exploit social policy for nationalist bio-politics, embedded in the realisation of the race-based eugenic-state. In addition, the establishment of the *Kassenärztliche Vereinigung* further co-opted physicians and their professional organisations into the Nazi-state.[51]

Additional political interventions in 1936 had an enormous impact on hospital funding. Until then hospitals had been increasing daily rates to finance rising expenses. As a consequence, public spending for hospital treatment continued to rise. The so-called Price-Stop-Decree (*Preis-Stopp-Verordnung*) fixed prices for medical care and treatment and was not rescinded until 1948. Furthermore, as part of the enforced political co-optation affecting all fields of medicine, the so-called monistic principle of hospital funding had been implemented. Heretofore, hospitals had been free to enter into contractual arrangements with private persons, insurance funds, and municipalities (or federal states) and could subsidise the construction of new buildings or expensive equipment (beside budgeting deficits). But the new law stipulated that all income had to originate from *one* single (monistic) source. The duration of a patient's hospital stay was calculated using a centrally fixed daily rate that took into account expenses for food, staff and maintenance; and medical treatments were calculated using a fixed expense ratio and the sum for care and cure billed to (and financed by) the patient's health insurance fund. In principle, hospitals' income from health insurance funds had to cover all of their costs (*Selbstkostendeckungsprinzip*).[52] Medical schools were able to apply to the Ministry of Education for extra money to pay for scientific equipment and expenses related to teaching.

The monistic principle also affected direct payers. In 1936, self-employed individuals or those with high levels of income (above the assessment ceiling and thus exempt from social security contributions) could pay hospitals directly. But with the implementation of the monistic principle this was no longer possible, forcing these individuals to insure themselves in so-called private medical insurance funds.[53]

The so-called monistic principle represented the starting point of direct state intervention and regulation of hospital organisation: hospitals were obliged to enter into contracts; prices for care and medical treatment were fixed; health care administrators centrally planned the supply of hospital beds and the construction of hospitals (*Krankenhaus- und Bettenbedarfsplan*); and hospitals were financed solely by statutory or private health insurance funds. This led to two main problems for the future. Although regulated by the state, hospital funding remained difficult, especially during the war.[54] In addition to implementing general cost reduction programmes, hospital administrators tried to compensate for deficits and funding shortfalls by suspending maintenance work or deferring necessary capital investments. Second, hospitals became dependent on health insurance funds as their sole source of revenue, a problem which, as we shall see, preoccupied administrators for decades to come.

Hospital funding in the post-war period through the late 1960s

During and after the Second World War, the entire welfare and health care system collapsed. On the one hand, the situation was similar to that after the First World War: wounded soldiers and invalids returning home needed urgent medical treatment, infectious diseases like tuberculosis and deficiency diseases drove a steady stream of patients into already overcrowded hospitals, while at the same time one third of the health care infrastructure, including hospitals, had been damaged or destroyed.[55] On the other hand, everything remained unchanged: hospitals were generally operated by municipalities (92%) and to a lesser extent by churches (5%) and private owners (3%); hospital fees were still fixed at 1936 levels and the monistic system of financing continued. In the initial chaos of the post-war era, hospitals complained that financial restrictions prevented them from guaranteeing proper care and cure. In June 1948 price controls ended on medical services and daily hospital rates (*Preis-Freigabe-Anordnung*). But in response, a couple of months later, health insurance funds complained that without price controls, they would go bankrupt. And so again, rates for daily care and medical treatment were fixed, but this time at a higher level than before (*Pflegesatzanordnung*).[56]

After the currency reform and the foundation of two different German states, further adjustments became necessary in West Germany. There, in September 1954, the government passed a law implementing rules on hospital fees.[57] Subsequently, a commission consisting of members of the health insurance funds, hospitals and civil servants from the Federal

Health Office and later from the Federal Ministry of Health negotiated the daily rates and fees for medical treatment and regularly adjusted them to account for inflation.[58]

The implementation rules stipulated that hospital fees cover the institution's own operating costs (*Selbstkosten*), including food, accommodation, medical treatment and basic maintenance. Marie-Theres Starke has shown that the term *Selbstkosten* meant different things depending on whether an institution was a charitable or a business enterprise: in the fee schedules of charitable institutions there was no accounting for profits or for interest rates on equity capital. But more importantly, there was no provision for long-term capital investments in larger medical devices nor for the construction or restoration of war-ravaged physical plant.[59]

De facto, the daily rates led to an under-funding of health care institutions. Ultimately, deficits had to be covered by hospital owners or bank loans. Analysing the long-standing structural causes of the deficits, Starke pointed to the charitable origins of hospital financing which had tended to separate donations for land and buildings and the overall planning of bed-capacities from the hospital's ongoing fee-based economy and operating costs.[60]

In the context of these concerns, health insurance funds played an ambiguous role. Like hospitals, they too were part of the commission charged with negotiating health care fees. But since hospitals' main source of revenue was derived from patient fees paid for by health insurance funds, the funds had no interest in higher fees. Moreover, neither the funds themselves nor anyone else believed they should be responsible for constructing hospitals or promoting technical innovations. In addition, the West German government was loath to increase the health insurance rates in order to finance the modernisation of hospitals. Government officials feared that rising health insurance contributions would increase labour costs and threaten the competitiveness of Germany's still fragile post-war economy.

All of this points to a fundamental problem of the monistic principle of hospital funding in twentieth-century Germany: hospitals' dependency on health insurance funds as their sole source of income exposed them to the interests of employers and employees and tied their financial wherewithal to the vagaries of the market economy. Economic recessions forced hospitals do draw on their reserves, resulting in technical equipment and hospital buildings (much of which dated back to the 1930s or the turn of the century) becoming outdated in the 1950s and 1960s. Physicians complained about inadequate equipment and about German medical science falling behind international standards.[61] As early as the 1950s, contemporary concerns about the investment backlog led to renewed calls by politicians and health care policy experts for a reform of hospital funding.[62]

The following discussion focuses on West Germany for two main reasons. At first, the development and problems of hospitals as such in West and East Germany were quite similar until the 1960s. Franz Knieps and Hartmut Reiners have concluded that, due to deferred investments, there was little difference between hospitals in West and East Germany until the 1970s.[63] And second, the system of hospital funding and the debates about lacking money, beginning in the 1960s in West Germany, continued onwards in the 1990s in the unified Germany. Nevertheless, it has to be mentioned that the funding of hospitals in East Germany was quite different. Social security and the health sector, and hospitals as part of it, were financed partly by workers' and employees' social security contributions, organised and administrated by the Free Federation of German Trade Unions (FDGB) and by direct state subsidies. According to the type and size of a hospital, the money was re-distributed using centralised expenses- and bed capacity-plans. Booklets about health economics and hospital funding published mainly undifferentiated figures about increasing amounts of money successfully spent on health and hospitals. Thus, complaints about crumbling buildings, lack of medicine and out-dated equipment were not discussed in public as in West Germany, though people could write petitions to governmental authorities, asking for instance for additional medicine or specific medical treatments.[64]

The shift from monistic to dualistic funding in the early 1970s

In the 1960s, several attempts were undertaken to reform the system of hospital funding in West Germany, which by 1966 had seen hospital deficits balloon to 1.355 billion marks. The Federal Minister for Employment drafted two bills—both of which were opposed by various interest groups and ultimately rejected—and created a commission with the task of evaluating the effectiveness of the social security system.[65] The Ministry of Health, headed by Elisabeth Schwarzhaupt, created another commission tasked with evaluating the hospitals' financial situation, their demand for new buildings and their need for new technical investments. This commission's report, the so-called Hospital Enquête of 1969, concluded—not surprisingly—that the existing structure did not ensure adequate medical care for the population and that hospitals produced an annual deficit of between 800 million and two billion marks.[66] The commission's suggestions were included in a new law that came into effect in June 1972: The Hospital Funding Law (*Krankenhausfinanzierungsgesetz*).

The Hospital Funding Law represented a fundamental shift in the system of hospitals finance. It replaced the monistic funding structure with a so-called dual structure. Patient fees, charged and invoiced by hospitals to health insurance funds for the care and medical treatment of their members, remained a key source of hospital revenue. But the construction of new buildings, the modernisation of older ones and investment in new technical equipment were now financed directly by federal and state governments. Ensuring adequate health care infrastructure, especially a sufficient number of hospital beds, came to be defined as a public task.

The Hospital Funding Law sought to combine divergent aims. First, the law aimed to secure the economic viability of hospitals and put their finances on a sound footing. Second, the law was designed to ensure adequate health care for the general population. And third, these aims needed to be achieved within the framework of socially acceptable social security contribution rates. The dual funding structure sought to ensure, on the one hand, the modernisation of hospitals and medical care. On the other hand, state funding of capital investments was intended to ensure that social security and health insurance contributions would not increase and thus put German companies and the economy in general at a disadvantage in international competition.[67]

As a consequence of the new law, the investment backlog was eliminated and a decade of major investment in modern equipment and new buildings ensued. The state's commitment to investment in health care infrastructure occurred against the backdrop of a sea change in German politics. Until the end of the 1960s, liberal-conservative governments (Christian-Democrats in coalition with Liberals) focused on economic growth and a balanced budget. The Social Democrats joined the conservative government as junior partners in 1966 and in 1969 became the ruling party, changing the political landscape of West Germany.[68]

After the reconstruction of Germany and the 'economic miracle' of the 1950s and 1960s, Social Democrats embarked on policies of economic redistribution. Although the oil crisis pushed the West German economy into recession in 1973 and threatened to upend increased spending on health care infrastructure, Social Democrats embarked on a policy of deficit spending in hopes of stimulating the economy.[69] The money spent by the state on investments in hospital infrastructure tripled from one billion marks in 1972 to 3.5 billion in 1973, while expenses incurred by hospitals for treatment and care and paid for by health insurance increased from 9.4 billion marks in 1972 to 25.4 billion in 1980.[70]

Soon, conservative politicians and health insurance funds complained about skyrocketing costs in the health care sector, predicting the system's imminent collapse. New technical devices and large-scale equipment (like computer tomography and magnetic resonance imaging), and the computerisation of medical diagnostics helped to drive costs upward. In general, the costs of medical treatment and care rose and health insurance funds accrued debts which they tried to compensate by raising health insurance contributions from 14% of earned wages (half of which was paid by the employer and half by the employee) in 1967 to 19.2% in 1985. In the mid-1970s, the Christian Democratic Minister of Social Affairs in the state of Rhineland-Palatinate, Heiner Geißler, warned that the total expenditure for health care was on track to triple and the employee's health insurance contribution would increase from 8.1% to 13.1% of earned wages. In this context, Geißler introduced the politically controversial and polemical term "cost explosion" (*Kostenexplosion*).[71]

In addition to expansive and expensive investments, other aspects of the Hospital Funding Law were also subject to scrutiny in the 1970s. Critics lamented the lack of effective cost control mechanisms and complained that hospitals were wasting public money. In general, more and more voices raised doubts about whether hospitals were a public good and the public's responsibility, reinvigorating claims that hospitals produced marketable services just like other enterprises.[72] Furthermore, since 1972 the federal government had calculated the demand for hospital beds centrally in an effort to overcome the backlog in infrastructure investment. Since these investments also affected the outlays of the federal states (which were responsible for a portion of the infrastructure spending), the states now criticised the federal government's mismanagement and demanded a greater role in decision-making processes.[73]

In an effort to put the genie of rising costs back into the bottle, the German parliament adopted a law in 1977 designed to reduce expenditure on medical treatment, but the law had little impact and was followed by another in 1981 designed to cut back on the benefits provided by health insurance funds.[74] In contrast with earlier efforts, the 1970s heralded the beginning of an era of ongoing health care reform. As each reform agenda was enacted into law, another would follow to offset the problems created by the preceding legislation.

Restructuring hospital finance since the 1980s

In 1982, a new conservative-liberal government assumed power and tried again to rein in rising expenditure on hospitals and health care. In December 1984, a new reform bill restructuring hospital planning and finances passed the parliament (*Krankenhaus-Neuordnungsgesetz*). Henceforth, two principles of hospital finance and accounting changed. First, the responsibility for hospital planning and finance passed from the federal government to the states. As a result, tariffs for care and cure were no longer centrally mandated by the federal government, but negotiated between hospitals and local health insurance funds.[75] The second involved cost management and was designed to counter accusations that hospitals wasted public money. Prior to the new legislation, hospital accounting was governed by an ex-post principle: it was not until the end of a patient's hospital stay that the various costs were calculated according to official tariffs and charged to the patient's health insurance fund. Thus, hospitals could generate income only when beds were occupied. This led politicians to insinuate that patients had been kept in hospitals longer than necessary and to complain that hospitals had no incentive to discharge patients earlier. In order to prevent this kind of malpractice, hospitals would in future have to calculate their occupancy rates in advance, as part of a national estimation (*Bettenbedarfsplan*), and based on this forecast hospitals were assigned a budget.[76] Another bill called the hospitals' charitable character into question by allowing them to turn a profit. It introduced a so-called flexible budget—meaning that savings from a previous accounting period could be transferred to the following period.[77] According to the neo-liberal *zeitgeist* of the 1980s, the aim was to allow hospitals that saved money to use it for other purposes, like research or technical equipment, while punishing the wasteful. Both laws implied a break with the long-standing principles of total cost reimbursement and ex-post accounting.

During an initial transition period, prospective budgeting was easy since the budget only had to be submitted for the current year. But in subsequent years, it became more difficult because both the budget and prospective bed occupancy rates had to be submitted ex-ante for the previous year. The new budget principles caused numerous problems, mainly because of the divergence between estimated targets and real-life numbers. And some hospitals were better situated to deal with the new rules than others, for instance hospitals in regions with older populations or treating patients suffering from chronic diseases faced disadvantages compared to those in regions with a younger and healthier population. Because the treatment of some diseases, like hemolysis, dialysis or organ transplantations, was particularly expensive, just a few such patients in one hospital's district could wreak budgetary havoc. Beside these imbalances, hospital administrators complained about the increased bureaucratic burdens of the new accounting techniques.[78]

And yet, in spite of these changes, key problems remained unsolved. Declining rates of mortality and morbidity since the Second

World War were resulting in an older population with more chronic diseases. Patients and employers were becoming more demanding as rising health insurance contributions raised expectations about the quality of medical services. And as the health care system expanded, the growing influence of lobby groups, each in competition for resources, was not just making root and branch reforms more difficult, but also further transforming health care into a commodity with high profit margins, especially for pharmaceutical companies and manufacturers of medical equipment. All of these problems intensified after German unification in 1990 as East German hospitals were renovated and integrated into the West German system of hospital financing.

The hospital system produced a number of imbalances, such as the treatment of patients suffering from cost-intensive diseases, unpredictable increases in patient numbers (due to an epidemic or the closure of a nearby hospital), or an atypical age structure (in rural areas). In order to manage these imbalances, exceptions were clearly defined and cost-intensive diseases were allowed to be accounted for separately. Over time, ever more exceptions were made and in the 1990s the whole system was—again—revamped by a number of new laws.[79] The introduction of so-called case rates, as formulated in the 1993 Health Structure Law (*Gesundheitsstrukturgesetz*), superseded the calculation of daily rates for bed occupancy and represented another decisive shift in accounting practices. Accordingly, each disease was allotted a 'normal' number of occupancy days. If a patient with a certain disease was discharged earlier, the hospital made a profit; if the patient stayed longer, the hospital lost money. Overall, it was assumed that profits and losses would cancel each other out. But this mode of accounting caused numerous problems: what happened if a patient had been released too early or if complications arose? And what happened if a patient was transferred to another hospital? And again, this change did nothing to address the hospital financing system's main problems and contradictions: predicted treatment vs. actual treatment; targeted costs vs. actual expenses; fixed estimated costs vs. varying actual costs; projected vs. actual patient numbers; not to mention the fundamental contradiction between health as a commodity vs. health as a public good.[80]

Throughout the twentieth century the proportion of private clinics remained small. In 1991, a quarter of all hospitals (358 in relation to 2,050 in public and charitable ownership) were privately owned. Beside those owned by charitable foundations or the Red Cross, they often had only a small number of beds, were led or owned by consultants and offered special or alternative treatments—not covered by health insurance schemes. Other private clinics were sanatoria-like rehabilitations centres. But since the 1990s, after hospitals were allowed to make profits, some hospitals turned into commercial enterprises, some entrepreneurs already active in the health sector bought former municipal hospitals. Since the 1990s the number and size of these commercially operated hospitals has risen and even university clinics have been taken over (now 707 privately owned/commercially operated hospitals in relation to 1,244 in public and charitable ownership),[81] while the number of public, charitable and municipal hospitals decreased and a larger number of unprofitable hospitals were closed and overall the number of hospital beds decreased rapidly.[82]

In 2000, the new coalition government of Social Democrats and Greens reorganised hospital finances again and a number of structural reforms (the so-called *Gesundheitsreform*) were introduced, resulting in a variety of further state interventions.[83] These reforms drew on US accounting practices that posited a fictional calculation-unit "diagnosis" that was more detailed than the previous case rate. This "diagnosis"-unit became the new basis for the reimbursement of medical care and treatment. Hospital physicians now had to classify patients' diseases exactly, including (various) secondary diagnoses, as well as their healthiness. The amount that health insurance funds were charged for a patient's treatment depended upon that patient's "Diagnosis Related Group" (DRG). The detailed classification according to the DRG was designed to minimise the gap between ex-ante forecasts and actual results. But it involved immense administrative efforts—and in the end, the problems remained unresolved.[84] Furthermore, case rates and other success-oriented accounting systems caused other problems. Cases were sometimes diagnosed differently, for instance a normal delivery was less expensive than an abdominal delivery (C-section). The problem arose that doctors began choosing more expensive alternative therapies: the rate of C-sections increased rapidly in the 1990s as did surgical operations for disc prolapses (instead of time-consuming physiotherapy). At the same time, patients were discharged much earlier than in the 1980s or as early as possible and often patients were transferred to short-term nursing facilities (which they had to arrange and pay for themselves) or discharged so early that medical complications arose.

Conclusion

In general, there are three historical eras of hospital funding distinguishable in Germany. Prior to the 1930s, nearly anything was possible: in a pluralistic field, various actors were involved in negotiating tariffs and hospitals had different sources of income and the freedom to contract out their services. Between 1936 and 1972 hospital funding was characterised as monistic: hospital revenue was derived solely from (private and statutory) health insurance funds for medical services rendered to their members. In 1972, the monistic structure of hospital funding was transformed into a dualistic one: health insurance funds reimbursed hospitals for medical services and the state financed buildings and technical infrastructure.

In this chapter, I suggest a fourth historical phase, starting in the mid-1980s and characterised by permanent hospital finance reform, by continuous state intervention (and corrections) and by the conviction that neoliberal incentives and reward systems could reduce hospital costs. During this fourth phase, the notion of public health as a common good was replaced by the neoliberal notion of health as a commodity. Since the 1980s, hospitals have been able to either (rarely) turn profit or (more often) record losses. As a result, hospitals tried to find other sources of income, reduced their labour costs, merged, or closed. In rural areas, where hospitals had to provide less densely populated areas with an older population, politicians complained about lacking hospitals and insufficient health services. Paradoxically, since the 1990s the health industry has been identified as an important stimulus to the national economy and health economists have enthusiastically debated the commercial and economic potential of the health care market. At the same time, however, those same economists have criticised rising costs in the health care sector (and hospitals as indirect consumers of medical products).

In the 1920s, health insurance funds became the most important, and in the 1930s the only, funding source for public hospitals in Germany. This caused various problems. First, statutory health insurance had been established originally as an insurance programme for industrial workers. As further groups came to be included in the programme, health insurance funds began to contribute the lion's share of revenue for hospitals that served the medical needs of all groups of the population. Furthermore, hospital income depended on the national economic well-being because the funds' contributions were paid by employers and employees. During recessions funds collected fewer contributions and came under increasing pressure to save money. Furthermore, the financial situation of hospitals hinged on other expenses such as those for practitioners or drugs. If the overall cost of drugs rose, hospital finances were also indirectly affected because insurance funds were under pressure to save money. The fixed income of hospitals explains why German manuals on hospital economics focused primarily on bed capacity planning, expenditures, and, since the 1980s, efficiency.

The public image of hospitals changed in the 1970s. Until then, they were considered to be welfare institutions and an important part of the infrastructure of a healthy society (which in turn was seen as a basis for a stable political order),[85] to be a public good, and to be icons of modernity and national economic strength. This changed in the 1980s under neo-liberal governments. Hospitals and other community tasks were re-defined merely as cost factors—like patients—or as entrepreneurial profit-centres.

But this latest phase in the development of hospital financing is confounded by at least four paradoxes. First, for a long time it seemed to be a consensus in Europe that hospitals were not profit-orientated businesses but public responsibilities. Hospitals that try to find new fields of income, offer more expensive services, or regard patients as sources of profit are liable to be criticised for unethical behavior. Second, within a fixed state-controlled environment that restricted their sources of income, imposed contractual obligations, and fixed the prices they could charge for their services, hospitals were forced to act like entrepreneurs. This led, thirdly, to the paradoxical situation that, under neo-liberal auspices, hospitals were defined as profit-oriented enterprises which at the same time had to draw up annually ex-ante cost and income plans and to justify deviations from the plan in ways reminiscent of socialist economic policies. Fourth, longer life expectancy and more sophisticated medical equipment has certainly led to rising expenditure in the health care sector. Ever since the 1960s, resources have been scarce and experts have been predicting the system's bankruptcy. But it is misleading to suggest that insufficient funding will persist merely because hospitals act like entrepreneurs. In the end, hospital financing seems to have been played as a zero-sum accounting game: money saved at one hospital was missing at another, a surplus in one period was a loss in another, and a short term profitable strategic advantage at one juncture could become a costly disadvantage at another. Through it all, enormous resources of time and money have been eaten up by endless reforms to an immense administrative accounting system.

Acknowledgements

This book chapter is part of a broader project on accounting and bookkeeping in medicine in Germany and Britain between 1750 and 1950. I would like to thank Alfons Labisch, Fritz Dross, and the editors of this volume for their comments and advice on earlier versions of the chapter.

1. In addition to countless articles in newspapers and magazines (the news magazine Der Spiegel, for instance, had a thematic issue [No. 50] in 1970 titled: Is the hospital broke [Ist das Krankenhaus pleite?]), there is an overwhelming amount of literature lamenting insufficient funding and health care infrastructure. For example, for the 1960s, see Max Kibler, Das kranke Krankenhaus. Heilkunde im Spiegel unserer Zeit [The Sick Hospital] (Stuttgart: Hippokrates Verlag, 1962); for the 1970s, Harald Clade, Das kranke Krankenhaus. Reform der inneren Struktur [The Sick Hospital. Reform of its Inner Structure] (Köln: Deutscher Industrieverlag, 1973); for the 1980s, Thomas Dersee and Stephan Dupke (eds), Bankrott der Gesundheitsindustrie. Eine Kritik des bestehenden medizinischen Versorgungssystems [Bancruptcy of the Health Industry] (Berlin: Verlagsgesellschaft Gesundheit, 1981) and Ernst Bruckenberger, Dauerpatient Krankenhaus. Diagnosen und Heilungsansätze [Permanent Patient Hospital] (Freiburg: Lambertus, 1989). See also the various yearbooks Krankenhaus-Report [Hospital Report], including such thematic issues as Krankenhausversorgung in der Krise? [Crisis of Hospital Care?] in 2010 and Strukturwandel [Structural Change] in 2015. Such pessimistic views have also been adopted in the historical literature. See for example the preface in Alfons Labisch and Reinhard Spree (eds), Krankenhaus-Report 19. Jahrhundert. Krankenhausträger, Krankenhausfinanzierung, Krankenhauspatienten (Frankfurt: Campus, 2001) or the concerns about the decline of the German welfare state in Gabriele Metzler, Der deutsche Sozialstaat. Vom bismarckschen Erfolgsmodell zum Pflegefall (Munich: Deutsche Verlags-Anstalt, 2003).

2. See for instance the implementation of the West German government's hospital enquête [Krankenhaus-Enquête] in 1969, the commission on hospital finance [Kommission Krankenhausfinanzierung] of the Robert Bosch Foundation dating from the early 1980, and various commissions in the 1990s on structural changes and health reform (Gesundheitsreform). On the reform efforts, see Douglas Webber, 'Krankheit, Geld und Politik. Zur Geschichte der Gesundheitsreformen in Deutschland', Leviathan. Zeitschrift für Sozialwissenschaft 16 (1988), 156-203; idem, 'Zur Geschichte der Gesundheitsreformen in Deutschland. II. Teil: Norbert Blüms Gesundheitsreform und die Lobby', Leviathan. Zeitschrift für Sozialwissenschaft 17 (1989), 262-300; Sebastian Bechmann, Gesundheitssemantiken der Moderne. Eine Diskursanalyse der Debatten über die Reform der Krankenversicherung (Berlin: edition sigma, 2007); Ingo Bode, 'Die Malaise der Krankenhäuser', Leviathan. Zeitschrift für Sozialwissenschaft 38 (2010), 189-211; Franz Knieps and Hartmut Reiners, Gesundheitsreformen in Deutschland. Geschichte – Intentionen – Kontroversen (Bern: Huber, 2015).

3. In contrast to Anglo-American countries, where the commodification of health and competition between physicians was part of the system, in Germany such commodification was sharply criticised. For a long time, health was instead regarded as a common state-regulated responsibility. Paul U. Unschuld has spoken here of a German Sonderweg. On this, and more generally on the commodification of health, see Paul U. Unschuld, Ware Gesundheit. Das Ende der klassischen Medizin (Munich: C.H. Beck, 2009); and Alexandra Manzei and Rudi

Schmiede (eds), 20 Jahre Wettbewerb im Gesundheitswesen. Theoretische und empirische Analysen zur Ökonomisierung von Medizin und Pflege (Wiesbaden: Springer VS, 2014).

4. See for instance the complaints about insufficient funds expressed by the former medical director of the Charité hospital in Berlin, Ernst Horn, Oeffentliche Rechenschaft über meine zwölfjährige Dienst-führung als zweiter Arzt des Königl. Charité-Krankenhauses zu Berlin nebst Erfahrungen über Krankenhäuser und Irrenanstalten (Berlin: Realschulbuchhandlung, 1818). And along similar lines a century later, see the reflections of the director in the Prussian Ministry of Cultural Affairs Otto Krohne, 'Die zunehmende Verteuerung unserer modernen Krankenanstalten und deren Ursachen sowie einige Vorschläge, ihr entgegenzuwirken', Ergebnisse und Fortschritte des Krankenhauswesens. Jahrbuch für Bau, Einrichtung und Betrieb von Krankenanstalten (Krankenhausjahrbuch) 2 (1913), 43-96.

5. See the review of Florian Gebreiter and William J. Jackson, 'Fertile Ground: The History of Accounting in Hospitals', Accounting History Review 25 (2015), 177-82.

6. See Martin Gorsky and Sally Sheard (eds), Financing Medicine. The British Experience since 1750 (London: Routledge, 2006).

7. See the contributions in Labisch and Spree (eds), op. cit. (note 1). For the Hubertus-Spital in Düsseldorf in the sixteenth century, see Fritz Dross, 'Their Daily Bread: Managing Hospital Finances in Early Modern Germany', in Laurinda Abreu and Sally Sheard (eds), Hospital Life. Theory and Practice from the Medieval to the Modern (Frankfurt: Peter Lang, 2013), 49-66. On early modern Nuremberg, see Ulrich Knefelkamp, Stiftungen und Haushaltsführung im Heilig-Geist-Spital in Nürnberg. 14.-17. Jahrhundert (Bamberg: self-publishing, 1989). On Franconian hospitals in the early nineteenth century, Eva Brinkschulte, Krankenhaus und Krankenkassen. Soziale und ökonomische Faktoren der Entstehung des modernen Krankenhauses im frühen 19. Jahrhundert. Die Beispiele Würzburg und Bamberg (Husum: Matthiesen, 1998). For hospitals in Berlin in the last third of the nineteenth century, see Jochen V. Pelz, Das Etatwesen der städtischen allgemeinen Krankenhäuser der Stadt Berlin um die Jahrhundertwende (1890-1900). Krankenhaus im Friedrichshain (8.10.1874), Krankenhaus Moabit (7.11.1882), Krankenhaus auf dem Urban (10.6.1890) (unpublished MD thesis: Free University Berlin, 1982). On nineteenth-century Munich hospitals, see Christian Scheffler, Das Krankenhaus Links der Isar zu München. Organisation und Finanzierung in den 1860er und 1870er Jahren (Herzogenrath: Murken-Altrogge, 1997).

8. See for instance Steffen Fleßa, Grundzüge der Krankenhausbetriebslehre, 2nd edn (Munich: Oldenbourg, 2010) and, regarding the history of hospital funding, esp. 132-42.

9. As a general overview, see Guenter B. Risse, Mending Bodies, Saving Souls. A History of Hospitals, (New York: Oxford University Press, 1999). On the German context, see Marie-Luise Windemuth, Das Hospital als Träger der Armenfürsorge im Mittelalter (Stuttgart: Franz Steiner, 1995).

10. On the idea of a strong state in (German) absolutism, cf. Ernst Hinrichs, Absolutismus (Frankfurt: Suhrkamp, 1986) and Heinz Duchardt, Das Zeitalter des Absolutismus, 3rd edn (Munich: Oldenbourg, 1998). Concerning the state's and municipal responsibility for public health care in Germany, see Calixte Hudemann-Simon, Die Eroberung der Gesundheit 1750-1900 (Frankfurt: S. Fischer, 2000), 43-50; and Fritz Dross, 'Health Care Provision and Poor Relief in Enlightenment and 19th Century Prussia', in Ole Peter Grell, Andrew Cunningham and Robert Jütte (eds), Health care and poor relief in 18th and 19th century northern Europe (Aldershot: Ashgate 2002), 69-111.On the role of medical police, see Bettina Wahrig and Werner Sohn (eds), Zwischen Aufklärung, Policey und Verwaltung. Zur Genese des Medizinalwesens 1750-1850 (Wiesbaden: Harrassowitz, 2003).

11. See the tables on expenditures in the chapters about Munich, Augsburg, Bremen and Mannheim in Labisch and Spree (eds), op. cit. (note 1); for Berlin, Pelz, op. cit. (note 7).

12. For Düsseldorf, see Dross, op. cit. (note 7) and for Würzburg, see Friedrich Merzbacher, Das Juliusspital in Würzburg. Vol. 2: Rechts- und Vermögensgeschichte (Würzburg: Oberpflegeamt der Stiftung Juliusspital, 1979). The proportion of income from interest amounted to 27 %. At the Municipal Hospital in Munich, income from foundations and charitable associations was 9 % in 1830 (in 1850 24 % and 7 %, in 1870 31 % and 1 %, in 1890 15 % and < 1 % respectively). See Andrea Wagner and Reinhard Spree, 'Die finanzielle Entwicklung des Allgemeinen Krankenhauses zu München 1830-1894', in Labisch and Spree (eds), op. cit. (note 1), 95-140, table 8, 117. At the Municipal Hospital in Augsburg, income from interest in the mid-1850s amounted to 30% (foundations/charities and donations comprised altogether 5%). See Willi Langefeld, 'Wie kann ein Krankenhaus Gewinn machen? Finanzierung und Betriebsergebnis des Allgemeinen Krankenhauses der Stadt Augsburg 1811-1914', in Labisch and Spree (eds), op. cit. (note 1), 141-177, table 6, 149.

13. For example, the Royal Charité Hospital in Berlin received tributes from its estate Prieborn. See the hospital's budget files at Humboldt University Archive, Charité Direktion (henceforth HUA CD), No. 35; for privileges, see the budget files for 1800 in HUA CD, No. 1354-5.

14. In the 1850s 11% of the overall budget of the Community Hospital in Augsburg was derived from the municipality. Cf. Langefeld, op. cit. (note 12), table 6, 149. At the Mannheim hospital, the proportion of subsidies varied in the late 1830s between 35% (1838) and 50% (1835). See Nils Gabler and Reinhard Spree, 'Die finanzielle Entwicklung des Mannheimer Krankenhauses 1835-1890', in Labisch and Spree (eds), op. cit. (note 1), 203-243, table 10, 227).

15. According to Reinhard Spree, 'Krankenhausentwicklung und Sozialpolitik in Deutschland während des 19. Jahrhunderts', Historische Zeitschrift 260 (1995), 75-105, table 1: 13-15% of Prussian hospitals in the 1880s were owned by the state, around 40% owned by municipalities, and 23% owned by the church or religious orders. The remaining fifth included other charitable foun-

dations, hospitals of provincial or district ownership, hospitals managed by workers or miners' associations and privately owned hospitals. An overview about the hospital's sources of income in Germany around 1900 provides table 3 in 93 (I: 6% donations, II: 28% subsidies, III-V: 64% charges, VI: 2% others).

16. In 1800, the Charité hospital in Berlin received 25,000 Reichsthaler income from subsidies and 9,173 Reichsthaler from patient charges. In the late 1880s, the relationship had completely changed: subsidies from the Prussian state amounted to 256,955 Marks, whereas the income from patient fees added up to 889,000 Marks, see the Charité budgets in AHU CD No. 1357 and the triennial Charité budget for 1888/1891 in the Secret Prussian State Archive (GStAPK), HA I, Rep. 76 VIII D, No. 260. Similar at the Community Hospital in Munich: in 1830 subsidies amounted to 38% (in 1850: 13%, in 1870: 10%, in 1890: 4%, also the income from interest decreased), and patient charges to 16% (in 1850: 51%, in 1870: 50%, in 1890: 80%), see Wagner and Spree, op. cit. (note 12), table 8, 117.

17. On the history of health and hospital insurance see Dross, op. cit. (note 10); for southern Germany see Folker Förtsch, Gesundheit, Krankheit, Selbstverwaltung. Geschichte der Allgemeinen Ortskrankenkassen im Landkreis Schwäbisch Hall, 1884-1973 (Sigmaringen: Jan Thorbecke, 1995); Kilian Steiner, 'Grenzen und Potentiale einer frühen Krankenversicherung am Beispiel der Ersten Münchner Krankenhausversicherung 1813-1832', in Labisch and Spree (eds), op. cit. (note 1), 69-94; Christian Lehmann, 'Das Stuttgarter Katharinenhospital während des 19. Jahrhunderts zwischen Krankheitskosten-Versicherungskasse und Gesetzlicher Krankenversicherung', in Labisch and Spree (eds), op. cit. (note 1), 179-201; and for northern Germany Barbara Leidinger, Krankenhaus und Kranke. Die Allgemeine Krankenanstalt an der St. Jürgen-Straße in Bremen, 1851-1897 (Stuttgart: Franz Steiner, 2000). More generally concerning social and political problems, see Ute Frevert, Krankheit als politisches Problem 1770-1880. Soziale Unterschichten in Preußen zwischen medizinischer Polizei und staatlicher Sozialversicherung (Göttingen: Vandenhoeck & Ruprecht, 1984).

18. On the establishment of a solidarity association for male and female urban servants in the Franconian cities Bamberg and Würzburg around 1800, see Brinkschulte, op. cit. (note 7); Leidinger, op. cit. (note 17) describes various health and hospital insurance schemes in the city republic Bremen in the mid-nineteenth century.

19. See Frevert, op. cit. (note 17); see Dross, op. cit. (note 10); and Ernest P. Hennock, The Origin of the Welfare State in England and Germany, 1850-1914. Social Politics Compared (Cambridge: Cambridge University Press, 2007). Then as now, the German Statutory Health Insurance had been described as a role model for other states, see Gerhard A. Ritter, Sozialversicherung in Deutschland und in England. Entstehung und Grundzüge im Vergleich (Munich: C.H. Beck, 1983); Ernest P. Hennock, British Social Reform and German Precedents. The Case of Social Insurance 1880-1914 (Oxford: Clarendon Press, 1987); for the US, John E. Murray, Origins of American Health Insurance. A History of Industrial Sickness Funds (New

Haven: Yale University Press, 2007), 37-40.
20. See Förtsch, op. cit. (note 17), 17-30. Regarding the development and motives of the law, see Ritter, op. cit. (note 19), 28-41; Hennock, op. cit. (note 19), 155-165; Dross, op. cit. (note 10); Peter Rosenberg, 'The Origin and the Development of Compulsory Health Insurance in Germany', in Donald W. Light and Alexander Schuller (eds), Political Values and Health Care: The German Experience (Cambridge: MIT Press, 1986), 105-26; Florian Tennstedt, 'Die Errichtung von Krankenkassen in deutschen Städten nach dem Gesetz betr. die Krankenversicherung der Arbeiter vom 15. Juni 1883. Ein Beitrag zur Frühgeschichte der gesetzlichen Krankenversicherung in Deutschland', Zeitschrift für Sozialreform 29 (1983), 297-338; idem, Sozialgeschichte der Sozialpolitik in Deutschland. Vom 18. Jahrhundert bis zum Ersten Weltkrieg (Göttingen: Vandenhoeck & Ruprecht, 1981), 165-174; and idem, Sozialgeschichte der Sozialversicherung, in Maria Blohmke et al. (eds), Handbuch der Sozialmedizin. Vol. 3: Sozialmedizin in der Praxis (Stuttgart: Ferdinand Enke, 1976), 385-492. In 1884, 4.3 million people (or about 10% of the population) were insured, whereas today, according to the annual reports of the German Federal Ministry of Health, more than 72 million people (or 87% of the overall population) are insured.

21. The alternative health schemes and their effects are described for Bremen in Leidinger, op. cit. (note 17). Depending on the health insurance association, the number of days of lost income that were compensated and the length of hospital stays varied and was limited.

22. See Tennstedt (1983), op. cit. (note 20); Hennock, op. cit. (note 19), 155-165. On the creation of health insurance funds in Swabia, cf. Förtsch, op. cit. (note 17), 39-48.

23. In some German states the daily rate was set up (or approved) by the government. For Prussia, see Bernd J. Wagner, '"Um die Leiden der Menschen zu lindern, bedarf es nicht eitler Pracht": Zur Finanzierung der Krankenhauspflege in Preußen', in Labisch and Spree (eds), op. cit. (note 1), 41-68. Until the 1910s, smaller surgical operations, herbal medicine, baths or dressing of wounds might have been included. See Axel C. Hüntelmann, 'Economies of the Hospital', in idem and Oliver Falk (eds), Accounting for Health. Calculation, Paperwork and Medicine, 1500-2000 (Manchester University Press, 2021), 109-42.

24. Regarding processes of accounting at the Charité Hospital in Berlin Hüntelmann, op. cit. (note 23).

25. On twentieth-century health budgets, see Christopher Sirrs, 'The Health of Nations: International Health Accounting in Historical Perspective, 1925-2011', in Hüntelmann et al. (eds), op. cit. (note 23).

26. According to Albert Guttstadt (ed.), Krankenhaus-Lexikon für das Deutsche Reich (Berlin: Georg Reimer, 1900), IV, the number of hospitals in Germany rose from 3,000 in 1876 (140,900 beds) to 6,300 in 1900 (370,000 beds). In Prussia, the number of hospital patient per 10,000 inhabitants quintupled between 1846 and 1917, see Spree, op. cit. (note 15), 76-7. For Berlin, see Manfred Stürzbecher, 'Die Berliner Krankenhäuser 1886 bis 1967', Berliner Statistik 23 (1969), 75-81.

27. See Albert Frank, Die geschichtliche Entwicklung der gesetzlichen Krankenversicherung (unpublished MD thesis, Technical University Munich, 1994), 38-48. Ritter, op. cit. (note 19), 54. Ritter notes that at least 50% of the population had been included by 1913.

28. Soon after the foundation of health insurance programme, all parties started to build district associations to improve their negotiating position. On such efforts in Swabia, see Förtsch, op. cit. (note 17), 78-107. On the foundation of the Hartmannbund, see Eberhard Wolff, 'Mehr als nur materielle Interessen. Die organisierte Ärzteschaft im Ersten Weltkrieg und in der Weimarer Republik 1914-1933', in Robert Jütte (ed.), Geschichte der deutschen Ärzteschaft. Organisierte Berufs- und Gesundheitspolitik im 19. und 20. Jahrhundert (Köln: Deutscher Ärzte-Verlag 1997), 97-142; Gabriele Moser, Ärzte, Gesundheitswesen + Wohlfahrtsstaat. Zur Sozialgeschichte des ärztlichen Berufsstandes in Kaiserreich und Weimarer Republik (Freiburg: Centaurus 2011).

29. See also the published rates in Walter Albrand, Die Kostordnung an Heil- und Pflege-Anstalten. Zum Gebrauch für Ärzte, Verwaltungsbeamte etc. (Leipzig: H. Hartung & Sohn, 1903). The director of the Statistical Office in Düsseldorf discussed the need for comparative financial statistics in Otto Most, 'Städtische Krankenanstalten im Lichte vergleichender Finanzstatistik', Zeitschrift für Soziale Medizin, Säuglingsfürsorge und Krankenhauswesen sowie die übrigen Grenzgebiete der Medizin und Volkswirtschaft 5 (1910), 213-236. A fixed schedule of charges for practitioners was regulated by the state. See for instance the legal commentary on the 1924 schedule (which remained valid until the late 1940s) in Eduard Dietrich and Heinrich Schopohl (eds), Das Gebührenwesen der Ärzte und Zahnärzte. Preußische Gebührenordnung für approbierte Ärzte und Zahnärzte, Gebühren der Preußischen Medizinalbeamten, Reichsgebührenordnung für Zeugen und Sachverständige und Reichsversorgungstarif (Berlin: Richard Schoetz, 1927).

30. Cf. the dietary schedule "Beköstigungs-ordnung fur die allgemeinen Krankenanstalten der Stadt Düsseldorf 1923" and the tariffs "Aufnahmebedingungen und Kostentarif für die allgemeinen Krankenanstalten der Stadt Düsseldorf für 1923" in the Municipal Archive (Stadtarchiv StA) Düsseldorf, Dept. IV, No. 37792 and No. 37815, items 20–1.

31. See Ritter, op. cit. (note 19), 54 and table 1, 171 and Tennstedt 1976, op. cit. (note 20), 385-492.

32. See Krohne, op. cit. (note 4).

33. See the brochure in StA Düsseldorf, Dept. IV, No. 37792 and No. 37815, items 20–1.

34. See Florian Tennstedt, Soziale Selbstverwaltung. Vol. 2: Geschichte der Selbstverwaltung in der Krankenversicherung (Bonn: Verlag der Ortskrankenkassen, 1977).

35. Ironically, although the statutory health insurance programme was designed to diminish the influence of the Social Democrat Party, in fact, workers and employees, often party members, gained enormous influence.

36. For example, the number of sick-days or hospital-days were increased, the amount of daily sick-pay was increased, additional family members were insured, etc.

37. See Tennstedt 1976, op. cit. (note 20), 395-6. On health insurance funds in Swabia, see Förtsch, op. cit. (note 17), 159-67.

38. In Berlin and elsewhere in Germany, food shortages led to rioting, especially in the winter of 1917/1918. Reports on political conflicts between hospital management, physicians, left-wing workers' councils, and confessional nursing staff at the Charité in GStAPK, HA I, Rep. 76 VIII D, No. 26.

39. Inflation rates had already begun to rise during the war and increased to 40% in 1919, 239% in 1920, before finally exploding to 1,000% in 1922 and 10,000% in 1923. Inflation ended with the introduction of a new currency unit.

40. On the general problems afflicting public health care and hospitals at the time, see Detlev J.K. Peukert, Die Weimarer Republik. Krisenjahre der Klassischen Moderne (Frankfurt: Suhrkamp, 1987); Heinrich A. Winkler, Weimar 1918-1933. Die Geschichte der ersten deutschen Demokratie (Munich, C.H. Beck, 1993).

41. See the annual budgets in HUA CD Nos. 1389-95.

42. For the Charité, see the annual budget files in HUA CD Nos. 1390-8. For reports about lawsuits related to outstanding debts, see GStAPK, HA I, Rep. 76 VIII D, No. 26. And for an audit report initiated by the Prussian government in the early 1920s regarding deficit spending at the Charité, see GStAPK, HA I, Rep. 76 VIII D, No. 269.

43. Regarding ambulatories, see Tennstedt, op. cit. (note 34), 150-80.

44. Ambulatories were a source of bitter dispute between health insurance funds and medical associations, and within the medical profession between practitioners and health insurance-accredited doctors (so-called Kassenärzte). The conflicts revolved around issues like the oversupply of physicians (Ärzteschwemme), fears about lower physician pay and a so-called proletarianisation of physicians, patients' (free) choice of practitioners and hospitals, and medical associations' concerns about the 'socialisation' of health and medicine. Some of these concerns culminated in various so-called doctors' strikes, which saw practitioners refusing to accept health insurance certificates. Regarding the medical profession and the threat of out-patient facilities, see Peter Thomsen, Ärzte auf dem Weg ins 'Dritte Reich'. Studien zur Arbeitsmarktsituation, zum Selbstverständnis und zur Standespolitik der Ärzteschaft gegenüber der staatlichen Sozialversicherung während der Weimarer Republik (Husum: Matthiesen, 1996); Wolff, op. cit. (note 28); Moser, op. cit. (note 28).

45. AOK Düsseldorf to the Direction of the Municipal Hospital Düsseldorf, 7.8.1926, StAD, Dept. IV, No. 37810. On the situation of health insurance funds during the 1920s, see Walter Bogs, Die Sozialversicherung in der Weimarer Demokratie (München: J. Schweitzer, 1981).

46. Regarding discussions about rising expenditure, see Krohne, op. cit. (note 4). For

comparisons of the daily catering and cure rates of hospitals, see the correspondence about cost structures between the municipality of Breslau (now Wroclaw) and the Düsseldorf Municipal Hospital in 1926, and in general various tables comparing the daily rates of larger hospitals in Germany in the 1920s in StAD, Dept. IV, No. 37815. For published comparisons, see for instance 'Kurkosten-Tarife deutscher Großstädte', Zeitschrift für Krankenanstalten 21 (1925), Issue 2.

47. There is nearly no literature on private clinics in Germany. For Berlin, see Manfred Stürzbecher, 'Zur Geschichte der privaten Krankenanstalten in Berlin', Berliner Ärzteblatt 82 (1969), 114-27.

48. According to Franz Memelsdorff, 'Die Finanzgebarung der Krankenanstalten', in Julius Grober (ed.), Das Deutsche Krankenhaus. Handbuch für Bau, Einrichtung und Betrieb der Krankenanstalten, 3rd edn (Jena: Gustav Fischer, 1932), 866-905, especially 892-3, before the First World War 40% were insured, 30% were direct payers, and 30% had their expenses covered by welfare agencies. At the end of the 1920s, hospitals in Berlin received 57% of their income from health insurance funds, 6% from direct payers, and 37% from welfare agencies. After 1930, some of the funding from welfare agencies was assumed by health insurance funds.

49. The Law for the Restoration of the Professional Civil Service in April 1933 led to the dismissal and retirement of civil servants (including medical officials) who were of non-Aryan descent or who did not share the Nazi's political views. Several by-laws limited the ability of lawyers or physicians to hold public or semi-public positions or to be health insurance employees or contractors. On these issues, see Martin Rüther, 'Ärztliches Standeswesen im Nationalsozialismus 1933-1945', in Jütte (ed.), op. cit. (note 28), 143-193, esp. 148. Staff in local health insurance offices were especially prone to be dismissed for political reasons, and on average some 30% were in fact dismissed. See Tennstedt 1976, op. cit., 405-6.

50. To this day, health maintenance organisations are banned from the health care market in Germany. See Fleßa, op. cit. (note 8), 132.

51. See Rüther, op. cit. (note 49). Regarding the ban of Jewish physicians, see Stephan Leibfried and Florian Tennstedt (eds), Berufsverbote und Sozialpolitik 1933. Die Auswirkungen der nationalsozialistischen Machtergreifung auf die Krankenkassenverwaltung und die Kassenärzte. Analyse, Materialien zu Angriff und Selbsthilfe, Erinnerungen (Bremen: Bremen University, 1980); idem, 'Health-Insurance Policy and Berufsverbote in the Nazi Takeover', in Donald W. Light and Alexander Schuller (eds), Political Values and Health Care: The German Experience (Cambridge: MIT Press, 1986), 127-84. At the same time, the autonomous self-governance of health insurance funds was dissolved. Committee members of the funds were no longer elected by members but appointed by the government; and the district and national associations were placed under state control. See Tennstedt, op. cit. (note 34), 150-80.

52. See Fleßa, op. cit. (note 8), 132.

53. The centralisation of insurance fund payments and the exclusion of private payments

effectively excluded Jewish physicians as well as patients from general hospitals. See Leibfried and Tennstedt (eds), op. cit. (note 51) and Rüther, op. cit. (note 49).

54. The central planning of hospital beds needs also to be interpreted in the context of the NS-government's preparations for war. As discussed below, hospital and other health care institutions placed a premium on the reduction of costs. One effect was that, for mental asylum patients unable to work, food ratios were (wilfully or otherwise) calculated far below minimum sustainable levels, thus condemning patients to death by starvation.

55. For an overview, see Stefan Kirchberger, 'Public-Health Policy in Germany, 1945-1949: Continuity and a New Beginning', in Donald W. Light and Alexander Schuller (eds.), Political Values and Health Care: The German Experience (Cambridge: MIT Press, 1986), 185-238; and Christoph Sachße and Florian Tennstedt, Geschichte der Armenfürsorge in Deutschland. Vol. 4: Fürsorge und Wohlfahrtspflege in der Nachkriegszeit 1945-1953 (Stuttgart: W. Kohlhammer, 2012).

56. See the Anordnung über Preisbildung und Preisüberwachung nach der Währungsreform, 25 June 1948, Gesetzblatt der Verwaltung des Vereinigten Wirtschaftsgebietes, 61. And on the decree revoking it, PR 140/48 dated 18 December 1948, see Marie-Theres Starke, Die Finanzierung der Krankenhausleistungen als Sozial- und Ordnungspolitisches Problem. Untersuchung über die Auswirkungen eines Übergangs zu Kostendeckenden Pflegesätzen im Krankenhauswesen der Bundesrepublik Deutschland (Münster: Aschendorffsche Verlagsbuchhandlung, 1962), 28. The proportional distribution of hospitals regarding their ownership in the Eastern parts of post-war Germany in W. Grossmann and H. Richau, Zur Ökonomik des staatlichen Gesundheitswesens in der Deutschen Demokratischen Republik (Berlin: VEB Verlag Volk und Gesundheit, 1962), 12.

57. Bundespflegesatz-Verordnung resp. Verordnung über Pflegesätze von Krankenanstalten, 31 August 1954, enforced 9 September 1954.

58. See Starke, op. cit. (note 56), 44. Michael Simon, Krankenhauspolitik in der Bundesrepublik Deutschland. Historische Entwicklung und Probleme der politischen Steuerung stationärer Krankenversorgung (Opladen: Westdeutscher Verlag, 2000), 41-57. Joachim Wiemeyer, Krankenhausfinanzierung und Krankenhausplanung in der Bundesrepublik Deutschland (Berlin: Duncker & Humblot, 1984), 19, has remarked that the proportion of hospital expenses in relation to the total amount spent by health insurance funds decreased from 19.23% in 1950 to 16.48% in 1960.

59. See Starke, op. cit. (note 56), 45-6.

60. See Starke, op. cit. (note 56), 22-3, 28. In the nineteenth century, publications dealt mainly with the construction of hospitals. From its first edition in 1910, the compendium Das deutsche Krankenhaus contained large chapters on the construction and funding of new buildings, in addition to chapters on hospital finance in general. This tradition continued in manuals on hospital economics published in the 1960s, for instance the standard reference (published in various

editions and still in print) of Siegfried Eichhorn, Krankenhausbetriebslehre. Theorie und Praxis des Krankenhausbetriebes, 2 vols., (Stuttgart: W. Kohlhammer, 1967 and 1971). Two chapters deal with bed capacity planning, funding and construction of buildings (altogether 21-158), and two separate chapters deal with accounting and hospital finance.

61. The public discussion is summarised by Wiemeyer, op. cit. (note 58), 21-4.

62. Starke's work, op. cit. (note 56), contributed to this discussion. She suggested budgeting for building maintenance and raising health insurance contributions. The reform of hospital funding was only one of various other issues in discussions about the reform of statutory health insurance. See Ursula Reucher, Reformen und Reformversuche in der gesetzlichen Krankenversicherung (1956-1965). Ein Beitrag zur Geschichte bundesdeutscher Sozialpolitik (Düsseldorf: Droste, 1999).

63. See Knieps and Reiners, op. cit. (note 2), 79-80. Also Helmuth Jung, 'Political Values and the Regulation of Hospital Care', in Donald W. Light and Alexander Schuller (eds), Political Values and Health Care: The German Experience (Cambridge, MIT Press, 1986), 289-324, concludes, that "normative and financial controls [of hospital care] in the two German states were remarkably similar" (p. 289).

64. As an overview see Grossmann and Richau, op. cit. (note 56), Hartmut Rolf, Sozialversicherung oder staatlicher Gesundheitsdienst? Ökonomischer Effizienzvergleich der Gesundheitssicherungssysteme der Bundesrepublik Deutschland und der Deutschen Demokratischen Republik (Berlin: Duncker & Humblot, 1975); Herbert Mrotzeck and Herbert Püschel, Krankenversicherung und Alterssicherung (Opladen: Leske + Budrich, 1997), part A; and Alfred Keck (ed.), Planung und Ökonomie des Gesundheitswesens (Berlin: Verlag Die Wirtschaft, 1981); on petitions as a form of protest and a way to deal with deficient medical supply in the East German health sector see Florian Bruns, 'Krankheit, Kon-flikte und Versorgungsmängel. Patienten und ihre Eingaben im letzten Jahrzehnt der DDR', Medizinhistorisches Journal 47 (2012), 335-367.

65. On the call for a reform of hospital funding, Knieps and Reiners, op. cit. (note 2), 79.

66. Estimates of the deficit varied depending on the mode of calculation. See Wiemeyer, op. cit. (note 58), 20-1 and Albert Holler, 'Das Finanzierungssystem nach dem Krankenhausfinanzierungsgesetz (KHG) und Fragen der Versorgungseffizienz', in Christian Ferber et al. (eds), Kosten und Effizienz im Gesundheitswesen. Gedenkschrift für Ulrich Geißler (Muinch: R. Oldenbourg, 1985), 153-166, 158. In total, expenditure on hospitals added up to some eight billion marks in 1969.

67. Holler, op. cit. (note 66).

68. For an overview, see Axel Schildt, Die Sozialgeschichte der Bundesrepublik bis 1989/90 (Munich: R. Oldenbourg, 2007); idem and Detlef Siegfried, Deutsche Kul-

turgeschichte: Die Bundesrepublik – 1945 bis zur Gegenwart (Munich: Hanser, 2009); Eckart Conze, Die Suche nach Sicherheit. Eine Geschichte der Bundesrepublik Deutschland von 1949 bis in die Gegenwart (Munich: Siedler, 2009).

69. See Schildt, op. cit. (note 68); idem and Siegfried, op. cit. (note 68); Conze, op. cit. (note 68).

70. See Holler, op. cit. (note 66), 159.

71. See Knieps and Reiners, op. cit. (note 2), 81. They note that Geißler's prognosis was distorted because he indexed expenses beginning from the relatively low baseline of 1960.

72. See Wiemeyer, op. cit. (note 58), 90-1. Thirty years later, health care was unquestionably deemed a marketable good. See Knieps and Reiners, op. cit. (note 2), 81.

73. See Wiemeyer, op. cit. (note 58), chap. II.

74. On the Krankenversicherungs-Kostendämpfungsgesetz (Medical Insurance Cost Containment Bill) of 1977 and the Kostendämpfungs-Ergänzungsgesetz and Krankenhaus-Kostendämpfungsgesetz (Supplementary Cost Control Bill and the Hospital Cost Control Bill) of 1981, see Fleßa, op. cit. (note 8), 134 and the Bundesgesetzblatt 1977, 1069 and 1981, 1568 and 1578. See also Simon, op. cit. (note 58), 89-105; Knieps and Reiners, op. cit. (note 2), 81-3.

75. See Bundesgesetzblatt I, 1716-22, §§ 6, 18.

76. See Fleßa, op. cit. (note 8), 134; Knieps and Reiners, op. cit. (note 2), 84-5; Werner Gerdelmann, 'Auswirkungen und Reform der Krankenhausfinanzierung', in Ferber et al. (eds), op. cit. (note 66), 167-184; Hubertus Müller, 'Die Neuordnung der Krankenhausfinanzierung – eine zwingende Notwendigkeit der Gesundheitspolitik', in Ferber et al. (eds), op. cit. (note 66), 185-200.

77. See Bundesgesetzblatt I 1986, 33-9, § 17. Both profits and losses remained on hospitals' books.

78. On the reforms in the 1980s Webber, op. cit. (note 2), Bode, op. cit. (note 2), and Simon, op. cit. (note 58), 106-61.

79. These laws included the 1993 Gesundheitsstrukturgesetz (Law on health structure), the 1996 Stabilitätsgesetz (Law to stabilise hospital expenditures), the 1997 Krankenhaus-Neuordnungsgesetz (Law on the Re-Organisation of hospitals), as well as two other laws implemented in 1998 and 1999 by the new Social Democratic and Green Party coalition dealing with the stabilisation of hospital expenditures. See Fleßa, op. cit. (note 8), 133-5.

80. On the structural reforms in the 1990s, see Martin Pfaff and Dietmar Wassener, Das Krankenhaus im Gefolge des Gesundheits-Struktur-Gesetzes 1993. Finanzierung, Leistungsgeschehen, Vernetzung (Baden-Baden: Nomos, 1995); Knieps and Reiners, op. cit. (note 2), 231-6; Simon, op. cit. (note 58), chapter 4-6; Manfred Wiehl, 'Finanzie-rungsformen und Investitionsrechnung im Krankenhaus', in Dietrich Bihr et al. (eds), Handbuch der Krank-

enhaus-Praxis. Unternehmensstrategien für Praktiker (Stuttgart: W. Kohlhammer, 2001), 289-99; Dietmar Köhrer and Maik Beltrame, 'Entgelt- und Kalkulationssysteme', in Bihr et al. (eds), op. cit., 300-22.

81. In 2016, the three biggest operator Helios (H), Asklepios (A) and Sana (S) owned 112 (H), 102 (A) and 50 (S) hospitals with an annual turnover 5.8 (H), 3.211 (A) and 2.4 (S) billion Euros, treating 5.2 (H), 2.3 (A) and 2.2 million patients per year, see https://www.praktischarzt.de/blog/ranking-groesste-klinikverbuende (15 March 2019). For the figures of total hospitals in 1991 and 2016 see the Hospital Report, edited by the Federal Ministry of Health.

82. Between 1991 and 2016 the number of hospitals declined from 2,411 to 1,951 and in the same period the number of beds decreased from 640,000 in 1991 to 498,000 in 2016. On these figures, see the Hospital Report, edited by the Federal Ministry of Health.

83. Several laws were enacted to implement case rates (Fallpauschalengesetz 2002, Krankenhausentgeltgesetz 2003, and Fallpauschalenänderungsgesetz 2006) and diagnosis related case rates (2004). Additional laws implemented structural reforms, like the Statutory Health Insurance Modernisation Law (GKV-Modernisierungsgesetz) in 2003, the Hospital Finance Reform Law (Krankenhausfinanzierungsreformgesetz) in 2009 and the Hospital Structure Law (Krankenhausstrukturgesetz) of 2016.

84. See Karl Ernst Knorr, 'GKV-Gesundheitsreformgesetz 2000', in Bihr et al. (eds), op. cit. (note 80), 113-33; Knieps and Reiners, op. cit. (note 2), 265-74; Fleßa, op. cit. (note 8), 136-67 (especially regarding diagnosis-related case rates); and Leonhard Hajen et al., Gesundheitsökonomie. Strukturen – Methoden – Praxisbeispiele, 6th edn (Stuttgart: Kohlhammer, 2011), 173-214 and 286-348.

85. Cf. Frevert, op. cit. (note 17).

Chapter 4

The development of hospital systems in new nations: Central Europe between the Two World Wars[1]

Barry Doyle, Frank Grombir, Melissa Hibbard & Balázs Szélinger
(University of Huddersfield)

The study of hospitals has grown substantially in the last twenty years especially in Britain where there has been important work on issues of finance and control, particularly at a local level.[2] As this special issue shows, similar research is now underway in many countries, including France, Germany and Spain where the focus has been on the rise—or not—of a state-supported hospital system funded through compulsory state insurance.[3] Initial research tended to characterise pre-welfare state health provision as limited, disorganised and poorly funded while rarely recognising the significant development taking place.[4] Yet it is apparent that across much of Western Europe hospital provision was growing, with central and local state, philanthropy and the private sector all responsible for increased and improved services.[5] To fund this growth, a complex mixed economy of financial systems developed, including National Insurance, local authority funding, mutual insurance schemes and direct payments.[6] However, in all of these schemes access to hospital treatment was restricted while in terms of coverage the self-employed in business and agriculture were often excluded.[7]

Although studies of western European health care are growing, there is little published research examining the hospitals of Central Europe—a region dominated by emergent nations attempting to build new health systems from the ruins of Europe's old empires. The nations of central Europe fit uneasily into the traditions of the established nation state, their multinational roots and new nation status offering a very different perspective from which to view the development of their hospital provision.

To date, their hospital historiography has been dominated by a traditional medical history approach focused on individual institutions and specialties, often written by senior medical practitioners working at the hospital or in the area of specialism.[8] There have been important studies on the growth of hospitals in Czechoslovakia by Svobodný and Masova[9] and useful work on Poland,[10] though little critical analysis of the situation in Hungary.[11] The communist era in these countries imposed significant checks on historical method while history of medicine has been largely abandoned as a subject for medical degrees.[12] Much of the health history of the region before the Second World War has focused on racial policy, and especially eugenics, with major contributions from Paul Weindling and Marius Turda.[13] There is a more extensive historiography of the work of international agencies in these nations, with particularly rich research focusing on the Rockefeller Foundation,[14] including studies of support for health institutes, nurse training and the development of health policy generally.[15] However, the Rockefeller Foundation were not interested in the development of hospitals *per se*, although their field officers did amass a great deal of information on the establishment of national services in the 1920s.

Over the course of the interwar period the new nations of Poland and Czechoslovakia and a much-truncated Hungary sought to utilize health care, and especially hospital provision, as evidence of their progressivism and modernity and as a symbol of nationhood.[16] Yet their intentions were constrained by a complex health inheritance, persistent financial crises and significant health challenges, especially in their poverty stricken eastern regions.

Building on an understanding of the complex demographic, ethnic and economic structures this chapter will utilise case studies of Czechoslovakia, Hungary and Poland to examine the challenges faced by these new nations in delivering a modern health care system. It will explore three key themes: who provided hospitals and how did their scale and scope change over time? How and by whom were hospitals financed and how did this affect access? And did health care feature in the process of nation building? It will show that these three themes were linked as they were pursued by governments with the aim of providing more and better institutions, branded as the work of the new nation and underpinned by a seemingly modern, extensive payment system. Yet despite considerable effort, resource and political will, financial weakness, ethnic conflict and urban-rural divisions limited choices and curtailed the expansion and modernization of the institutional infrastructure.

Access to primary sources varied across the three nations. Both state and local records were extensive for Czechoslovakia, more limited for Hungary and almost non-existent for Poland, where the destruction of Warsaw and other major cities meant few public records survived.[17] The main sources utilised in this text are published reports, such as the *Czechoslovak Health Yearbook*, which provided extensive statistical material on provision and funding structures.[18] Similar, less full, publications exist for Hungary and Poland.[19] In the former case, extensive use has been made of medical and hospital journals for evidence of change at an institutional level and in all cases material has been drawn from insurance data. This has been supplemented by important national data collected by the League of Nations in the

1920s and the International Labour Organisation for the later 1930s. These surveys relied on local contacts well placed within the national health system and included both hospital statistics and information on the operation of insurance schemes.[20]

In a similar vein, the study has drawn on the international publication, *Nosokomeion*, which included a number of articles on general and specific issues concerning hospital services in Poland, Hungary and Czechoslovakia, with Poland receiving the most attention. In addition, particular use has been made of material from the Rockefeller Foundation who worked extensively in Central Europe in the 1920s. The Foundation appointed Selskar Gunn as a resident officer in Poland at the beginning of the decade and he continued to work closely with government health departments until the onset of the Depression saw a shift in RF focus away from Europe to Asia.[21] In addition to a collection of baseline country surveys conducted between 1920 and 1924 and ongoing field officer visits to the region, a number of local reports were produced by teams examining applications for Foundation grants. Together the RF material offers a rich mix of macro level assessment undertaken by policy insiders with considerable knowledge of the country and specific examples of health service provision on the ground.

The first section of this chapter will provide an overview of the health care, and especially hospital, inheritance of these nations at their formation in 1918 set in the context of demographic, ethnic and economic variables. The second will examine developments in the extent and ownership of hospital provision; the third explores the funding landscape, and how this affected access to care while the final section will consider the effect of the multi-ethnic character of these nations on the provision of hospitals and the role of health care in nation building.

The new geography of central Europe

Between 1918 and 1924, following the collapse of the German, Austro-Hungarian and Russian empires, a number of new or much re-drawn nations were created across central Europe.[22] Formed by local politicians and the peace treaties, these countries combined national self-determination with economic and geographical pragmatism, leaving multi-ethnic states to cope with recalcitrant minorities, unsatisfied neighbours, angry separatists and a substantial Jewish minority that the new countries only partially tolerated.[23] In this environment, the body was a key site for the legitimation policies of the new nations with eugenics, racial politics and health care strategies deployed to tie together the disparate national and ethnic groups.[24] In their quest for political legitimacy the governments of the new states directed some of their energies to the creation of modern, efficient and progressive health care provision, often using this to establish a sense of democratic entitlement and national identity.[25] Yet this was a difficult and complex task. Poland and Czechoslovakia inherited multiple hospital systems from their former imperial rulers; Hungary was massively reduced in size and lost many of its leading institutions to the successor states; each new state had large geographical areas with very limited service provision, especially in the eastern lands; and all had to deal with huge financial difficulties, including inflation, currency instability and the effects of the economic depression.[26]

The Polish Republic was created out of lands from each of the former empires including German Silesia and the Polish Corridor, Galicia from Austro-Hungary and both Congress Poland (the central area around Warsaw) and the Pale of Settlement, the predominantly rural area with a largely Jewish population, from Russia.[27] The background for Czechoslovakia was equally complex, with the Czech lands of Bohemia and Moravia in the west seceding from Austria, while Slovakia and Ruthenia were Hungarian territories, the latter with a substantial Jewish population.[28] As a result of the Treaty of Trianon (1920), however, Hungary saw its population and landmass reduced by almost 60%, with the large and urbanised region of Transylvania transferred to Romania while substantial territory was ceded to the new states of Yugoslavia and Czechoslovakia.[29]

This complex inheritance was important for a number of reasons. Although Hungary was reduced to a coherent ethnic and linguistic core by the peace settlement, elsewhere ethnic diversity led to problems with delivering a unified, national health system. In Czechoslovakia the Germans continued to maintain and guard their own provision, while in the cities like Prague the main hospitals and the medical schools operated on separate ethnic grounds.[30] In Eastern Poland, the geographical and economic limitations of the dispersed Jewish settlements demanded a different approach to institutional care to that found in the rest of the country.[31] As Table 1 shows, roughly one third of the population of Poland and Czechoslovakia belonged to another ethnic group, with Germans forming a powerful lobby in west Czechoslovakia and Ukrainians and Jews in Eastern Poland. This was particularly apparent in some big cities, with Poles a bare majority of the citizens of Lemberg/Lvov, while Jews numbered around a quarter of the population of Budapest.[32]

Table 4.1: Ethnic Population of Czechoslovakia, Poland and Hungary, percentage distribution, 1921-31

	Czechoslovak	Polish	Hungarian	German	Jewish	Other
Czechoslovakia (1921)	65.3	1.0	5.5	23.3	1.3	3.6
Poland (1931)	-	68.9	-	2.1	10	19
Hungary (1930)	1	-	92	2	5	-

Sources: Heimann, *Czechoslovakia*, 64-5; Prażmowska, *History of Poland*, 102; Molnár, *A Concise History of Hungary*, 268.

The first problem facing these new states was managing the effects of the First World War. In much of the region, especially across Poland, there was considerable war damage compounded by the ongoing disputes with Ukraine and Soviet Russia that lasted until 1922.[33] Millions of people were displaced in this process, some spending up to seven years away from their farms. Large numbers died in the fighting, or as a result of displacement or even of starvation in the famine that swept the region in 1920-21. Epidemic diseases were rampant, especially typhus, typhoid and recurrent fever, the latter proving more life threatening due to inadequate feeding. Around one and a half million houses had been destroyed, farms were in ruins with vegetation across the fields, there were no horses, implements, seed, timber or food and some returnees were reported to be living in the dugouts made by the German army.[34]

Though less extreme, in the Hungarian city of Gyär there were thousands of refugees from Transylvania living in overcrowded barracks while resources were diminished by looting, the occupying Serbian army stealing all of the operating theatre equipment of the small hospital in the southern town of Sikles.[35] The borders were officially settled by 1924, but disputes continued to cause instability in the region until 1939.

The economic effects of the treaty settlements hampered the growth of hospital systems. Economically these countries suffered many of the problems of other nations between the wars, but in an aggravated fashion. Both Hungary and Poland were plagued by hyper-inflation until major currency reform in the mid-1920s although the Czechoslovak economy remained stronger than the others and benefitted from a more stable currency.[36] Poland and Czechoslovakia were more economically advanced in the western regions ceded from the German and Austrian empires whose industrial and urban development was more extensive. However, in the eastern areas like Slovakia, Belarus and Subcarpathian Ruthenia (known by the Czechs as Podkarpatská Rus or PKR) subsistence agriculture predominated, there was little urban development and social infrastructure was limited.[37] For Hungary the loss of Transylvania and cities like Bratislava proved particularly problematic as they included many of the country's leading hospitals and medical schools. Moreover, outside of Budapest much of the country was rural, with few towns and a limited organisational base to support an extensive hospital system.[38] The later 1920s saw gradual expansion of public investment across the region, especially on hospitals. Thus, the Czechs focused on 'modernising' the east with public health projects in both Slovakia and PKR. In 1927, the Slovak politician in charge of health secured significant funding from the state insurance scheme surplus for infrastructure development in Ruthenia, including the continued upgrade of the hospital in Mukačevo.[39] However, these nations were badly hit by the depression leading to a significant squeeze on health spending.

All three nations had significant rural populations. In Poland roughly 75% of the population lived in the countryside, for Hungary the proportion was around 67%, while in Czechoslovakia the figure was over 40%.[40] Although there were urban centres in the west, especially in Bohemia and Polish Silesia, in central and eastern areas there were relatively few large towns and illiteracy was widespread, especially among the older population and women.[41] Transport and communications were weak and in parts of rural Slovakia and Poland the roads were impassable by cars. Moreover, some regions were very poorly integrated into the market. Currency was limited in the east of Poland, many peasants living within a barter economy—indeed there were attempts to allow payment for health services in goods rather than cash.[42] These problems were exacerbated in the early 1930s as the Great Depression forced down world agricultural prices, reducing incomes for farmers, workers and the state. Again, the effects were rather different in Czechoslovakia where both the industrial west and the rural east experienced recession at different points in the cycle and recovered at different rates. In all three countries state and local finances were severely affected, restricting both capital investment and operational income for health provision. However, recovery was driven, at least in part, by war preparation and rearmament and by the changes in relations with Germany after 1933.

There were, moreover, severe public health problems. Infant mortality was well above the western European average and remained stubbornly high throughout the period.[43] The lowest rates were found in Czechoslovakia where a steady decline was noted in the later 1920s to 140/1000 in 1929. However in Hungary the figure remained static at around 180/1000 while for Poland figures were only available for the more prosperous western and southern provinces where in 1926 the rate was 180/1000.[44] Across the region the infrastructure to tackle infant mortality, tuberculosis and contagious diseases was limited despite investment and support from bodies like the Rockefeller Foundation.[45] Mobile infectious disease units were developed for use in remote areas, especially PKR and eastern Poland[46] and across these regions the health centre—with the hospital as support—emerged as the key vehicle for delivering services.[47]

The new nations inherited a diverse range of health funding systems from the previous imperial regimes. The German, Austrian and Hungary governments had introduced health insurance by 1914, though this was absent from the Russian empire. Polish Silesia benefitted from the highly developed German system, established in the 1880s and offering cover to the region's industrial and white-collar workers. Austria was quick to follow Germany in establishing health insurance and by 1914 it covered a similar range of industrial and transport workers. In each case family members also benefitted. As a result, these two nations led the world in coverage in 1910 with around one third or more of the population insured by the end of the First World War. The new nations were quick to adopt and adapt these schemes, the Poles ambitiously basing their new national coverage on the German model (even if it was a largely unaffordable aspiration). Each nation also inherited the Hungarian system. Claimed to be the oldest in the world (a voluntary initiative was launched in the 1870s) a limited state health insurance scheme was in operation by 1891 covering a similar range of industrial and transport workers along with a wide range of state employees. In Russia, however, no compulsory state health insurance existed, leaving a substantial hole in the health finances of the new Polish state. Although these countries could draw on these existing schemes, significantly none of them included agricultural workers, a prominent part of each workforce.[48]

Hospital numbers

The new states inherited a health infrastructure based on the four different imperial systems. Hungary, Galicia, Slovakia and PKR had the Hungarian system with strong central control of local institutions. Bohemia and Moravia and Silesia had German or Austrian structures with a national insurance system but devolved hospitals. Poland had a complicated mix of all four former regimes and, with some good provision in the former Austrian, German and Hungarian areas although the bulk of the nation was covered by the very limited Russian inheritance with relatively few hospitals and a weak health infrastructure.[49]

Defining a hospital is a challenging exercise, especially in this period of rapid organizational, intellectual and technical change.[50] A basic definition might include any institution that accepts patients for residential treatment with the aim of curing or 'materially relieving' their condition. By 1918 the bulk of general hospitals had provision for surgery and internal medicine while increasing numbers had specialist departments for various parts of the body. They might include isolation facilities for infectious diseases, facilities to treat venereal diseases and in many cases maternity and gynaecology blocks. From the late nineteenth century specific demographic groups also secured specialist institutions, including women and children. But the hospital was also separating out traditional patient groups and developing services beyond the acute sector. Tuberculosis was usually treated separately from other infectious diseases. The elderly, the infirm and the chronically ill—the bulk of patients in the nineteenth century public hospital—were squeezed out, coming to occupy a less medicalised space in the hospice-style accommodation of the municipality.[51] Those with mental illnesses attracted their own, frequently overcrowded and underfunded, establishments. The extent of these divisions differed across Europe and North America and even within countries.[52]

Figure 4.1: Relative Proportion of Provision in Hospitals and Mental Institutions 1931

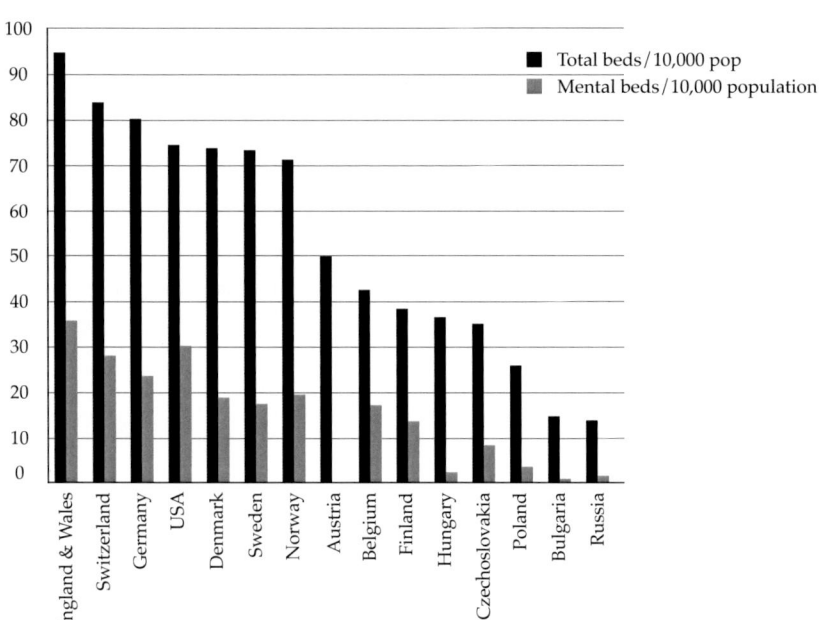

Source: C. Neville Rolfe, 'Hospital and venereal disease', *Nosokomeion*, 3, 3 (1932), 245. Total beds includes mental health beds.

The available statistics for central Europe, unlike those for the west, rarely distinguished between the curative general and specialist hospital and the care-oriented, chronic institutions associated with the hospice and the poor law.[53] Progress in the visible and politically important general teaching hospitals of urban centres can blind us to the lack of change in county areas administered by cash-strapped local authorities.[54] With these caveats in mind we can see the extent of hospital provision in Europe in 1931 (Fig.1). The northern and western European nations were offering a ratio of approximately 70-80 beds per 10,000 people while the Central European countries provided roughly half that number. But as can be seen from Table 2, progress was being made to increase capacity: first by building new institutions and, second, by renovating and reorganizing existing hospitals to meet modern demands—although many of these institutions still fitted the older model of mixed acute and chronic care, especially in rural areas.

Table 4.2: Number of Hospitals and Beds in Czechoslovakia, Hungary and Poland, 1918-37

	Czechoslovakia		Hungary*		Poland	
	Hospitals	Beds	Hospitals	Beds	Hospitals	Beds
1918	-	-	429	45,500	322	47,000
1920	163	26,000	183	26,500	-	-
1925	-	-	205	30,000	634	47,000
1930	389	53,500	233	40,000	656	53,000
1935	411	64,000	291	46,500	677	75,000

Sources: István Ágoston, *A kórházi kapacitások és szabályozásuk története*, University of Pécs, 2013, 104; Jiří Říha (ed.), Zdravotnická ročenka Československa, 1928-1940 (Vols. I-XI) (Praha: Piras, 1928-1940); Ministerstwo Opieki Społecznej, *Dwadzieścia lat publicznej służby zdrowia w Polsce odrodzonej, 1918-1938*.
* The figures for Hungary for 1918 show the number of institutions and beds prior to treaty changes.

In the case of Poland the key need was to increase the number and spread of institutions and in this there was success. When the new nation was formed in 1918 the country had just 332 hospitals with around 47,000 beds for a population of approximately 26 million.[55] The number and distribution of institutions improved significantly in the early 1920s while the mid-1930s saw a new programme of addition and improvement so that the hospital stock had reached almost 700.⁵⁶ From this point the number of institutions stabilized but capacity increased significantly while many of the smaller chronic hospitals that had dominated the countryside were upgraded to take more patients and adopt a more curative function.

The Czechoslovak Republic began with an inheritance of 163 hospitals and 26,000 beds in 1923 for a population of 13.4 million, or just over 2/1,000. By 1929, the number of hospitals and beds had almost doubled, while the period 1929-36 saw beds in general hospitals rise by almost a quarter and in all types of institution, including care-focused sick houses, they rose by a third from 70,000 to 93,000.⁵⁷

In 1918 the situation in Hungary was a little better than in Poland in terms of numbers of institutions and beds but as a result of the peace settlement, it lost 57% of its hospitals and 42% of its hospital beds. Yet the nation was able to overcome these problems and by 1935 the number of both had doubled so that there were more beds than in 1915 with a significantly higher ratio of beds to residents than before the War. Part of this transformation was the result of institutions built to replace those lost to neighbouring states, such as the Horthy Miklós Royal State Public Hospital at Debrecen opened in 1931 to serve the city and the new university.⁵⁸ In the following ten years over 100 additional establishments were added, restoring provision to above the 1918 level.

Along with deficiencies in the number of institutions these health systems also had to deal with the poor distribution of facilities, the interwar period seeing some progress towards a more uniform allocation. In post-war Poland the existing hospitals were unevenly distributed with virtually none in the north-east area along the Russian border, leading to the erection of 100 temporary hospitals in the region adding thousands of new beds. The average coverage also improved significantly to one bed per 467 inhabitants overall (just over 2/1,000) by 1938 but this was the national average; enormous regional disparities remained. For example, in the north east there was still only one bed for 1,250 persons and in the district of Postawski only one bed per 5,000 residents. Indeed it was calculated by the Ministry of Public Welfare that to meet the modern standard of three beds per 1,000 residents, beds would need to increase by around 50 per cent.[59] Similar uneven distribution in the quantity and quality of provision wa5s found in Czechoslovakia. For example, in 1920 the Czech lands (Bohemia and Moravia) possessed three quarters of the nation's hospital stock (123/163). Conversely there were just eight institutions in Silesia and four in Ruthenia, and these were all of very poor quality at this time.[60] The 1930s saw significant improvements in peripheral areas like Silesia, as well as attempts to modernize the under-developed region of PKR. Bed numbers in the region increased by 68% while the number of patients treated increased by 175%. However, this did cause problems as the facilities proved unable to keep up with the growth in demand and at Užhorod it was not uncommon for two or more patients to share a bed while others slept on the floor.[61]

As can be seen from Figure 2, new building in Hungary set out to address the poor distribution across the country. In 1923 Selskar Gunn had noted that: 'The total number of beds in the entire country is theoretically sufficient. However, the distribution is not the best, as Eastern Hungary is poorly supplied with hospitals' but by the later 1930s the east had secured a number of prominent new institutions.[62] Yet once again the distribution remained uneven with the central and eastern portions of the country less well served than the west and south. Moreover, the lost institutions were heavily based in Transylvania and included a number of medical schools as well as important hospitals. Replacements had to be established within the truncated Hungary in cities like Pécs (which acquired staff and equipment from the university at Bratislava), Szeged and Debrecen[63] supplemented by new hospitals in Budapest, like the Hospital of the National Insurance Institute, opened in 1927 with over 500 beds.

Figure 4.2: Hospitals in Hungary, 1938

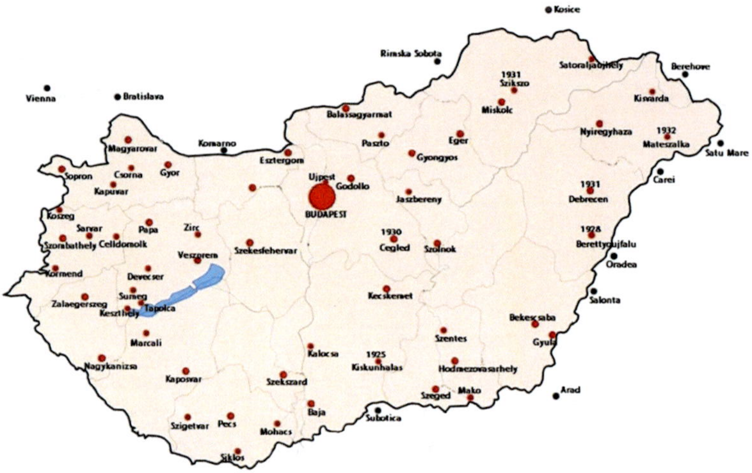

Map drawn by Balázs Szélinger.

Hospital Ownership and Management

In each of these three nations there was a mix of providers including central, regional and municipal government, charitable, philanthropic and private sector involvement.[64] Given their origins in the four predecessor systems, both Poland and Czechoslovakia even had more than one type of local provider. Thus hospitals in former Hungarian regions were managed by the higher level county authorities acting as the representatives of the central state, while in the Austrian areas the main provider was the lower tier city or district council—usually referred to as the municipality. This diversity was demonstrated by the Rockefeller Foundation's agent, Selskar Gunn, who found four main types of ownership in Hungary in 1923: a) state, b) public, c) semi-public, and d) private.

'A: State hospitals were run by central government and included university clinics, midwifery schools etc. The staff were well qualified civil servants. The fees were fixed by the Ministry.

B: Public hospitals were supervised by an Administrative Commission of the County and usually had departments of internal medicine, surgery and venereal diseases as well as accommodation for mental illnesses and infectious diseases. Fees fixed by Ministry of Welfare together with the county council.

C: Semi-public institutions were private hospitals recognized by the Ministry and therefore eligible for payments from public sources for treating the poor. Fees for sick poor set by Ministry in consultation with owners.

D: Private hospitals were subject to the supervision of the Administrative Commission but otherwise independent of the system.'[65]

Within categories C and D were to be found a number of religious institutions including the Brethren of Mercy.

These categories of ownership and responsibility were broadly replicated across the region, as shown by Tables 3 and 4, although in Czechoslovakia the private sector appears to have been weaker. Thus, in 1921, the largest number of hospitals in Hungary were private, including many run by religious houses, but these tended to be small or very small. The county hospitals, operating services for the central state, were the second largest category and they also included the bigger institutions, many with departments of internal medicine, surgery and venereal diseases, as well as accommodation for mental illnesses and infectious diseases. There was a relatively small number of medium-sized, semi-public hospitals recognized by the Ministry and therefore eligible for payments from public sources for treating the poor. In terms of specialist facilities, the biggest expansion, in line with developments across Europe, was among obstetrical clinics and hospitals which by 1930 numbered 34 and offered 4,700 beds. Counties were able to extend their hospital provision after 1928 with the assistance of US loans, almost 50 authorities taking advantage of the Speyer loans.[66] Thus, the Miklós Horthy public hospital in Nagykanizsa completed an extension funded by a combination of Ministry of Welfare loans and grants, a subvention from the County of Zala and over 600,000 pengo[67] from the town council thanks to a Speyer loan.[68]

Table 4.3: Hospital beds by type, Czechoslovakia 1921 (n. 163)

	Beds
Urban Hospitals (All)	8,967
District Hospitals (Bohemia)	7,672
State Hospitals (Bohemia, Moravia, Slovakia)	4,127
County Hospitals (Slovakia & Ruthenia)	2,186
Provincial Hospitals (Moravia & Silesia)	1,883
Private Hospitals (Not Ruthenia)	1,176
Total	26,000

Source: Pelc, *Organisation of the Public Health Services in Czechoslovakia*

In both Galician Poland and Slovakia, a similar pattern of provision was evident to that in Hungary of county management and state finance. In Poland the central state had limited input—mostly the infectious disease hospitals they had established in 1918. Generally local municipal control was the norm—although by the later 1920s federations of local authorities were joining together to build institutions of wider significance such as mental illness facilities. As can be seen from Table 4, by 1927 local government was the largest provider, although these were mainly small institutions, social organisations were very significant while the fully private sector was small in terms of beds. The social organisations included social insurance funds and social/congregational bodies, such as charities like the Red Cross, and religious and ethnic communities—Catholic, Jewish and Orthodox.[69] Among social insurance providers was Kasa Chorych, supported by very good hospitals in the west run by Spólka Bracka, the miners' insurance fund. In 1928 they ran eight hospitals, including the substantial, modern facility at Katowice which had undergone a significant extension, increasing capacity to just under 500 beds for internal, surgical, eye and ear patients.[70] The legacy institutions from the German and Austrian empires tended to be of a higher quality than those left by the Russians and Hungarians—although it was noted that the former German institutions were beginning to age by the later 1920s.[71] In the east, conversely, social insurance hospitals were less prominent, Bialystock did not have any kind of insurance institution until 1933.[72] However, there was an attempt in this region to meet need by the creation of health centres, supported by both the Rockefeller Foundation and by levies from the health insurance fund and offering preventive services and some mobile facilities.[73]

In general, the Public Health Department of the Polish Ministry of Welfare favoured a centralized system similar to that operating in Galicia, for it was seen to provide uniformity and financial stability.

In 1922 they had proposed taking all hospitals under state control and funding them as far as possible from state taxes.[74] However, many localities resisted this, claiming government preferred large, multi-purpose institutions rather than responding to specific local needs. Critiques of the 1928 Hospital Ordnance suggested it failed to support local initiative which had done much to develop hospital provision over the preceding fifteen years preferring urban new builds over improvement and better administration.[75]

Table 4.4: Hospitals in Poland by Provider, 1927 and 1937

Provider	No Institutions		No Beds	
	1927	1937	1927	1937
State	30	72	6,856	11,873
Local Government	343	283	31,433	37,659
Social Welfare Orgs	207	214	17,391	23,469
Private	76	108	1,633	1,971
Total	656	677	57,313	74,972

Source: Ministerstwo Opieki Społecznej, *Dwadzieścia lat publicznej służby zdrowia w Polsce odrodzonej, 1918-1938*

By 1937 there had been significant expansion of bed numbers especially in the facilities run by the state and the social welfare organisations, for example the Polish Red Cross. This was facilitated by increased state planning and a policy of closing hospitals with fewer than ten beds and, where possible, merging institutions to increase efficiency. For example in Suwalki, a town in northern Poland, the Hospital of St. Peter and Paul and the Jewish Hospital decided to merge since they already shared the same building.[76]

In Czechoslovakia a plan to nationalise the hospitals in 1920 only included a small number of strategic institutions, mainly in Prague leaving Hungarian-style county hospitals to operate in Slovakia and PKR and municipal control in Bohemia and Moravia. Private institutions were uncommon, although works' hospitals were common in the west, especially in the coal mining areas. However, the most famous company institution was the Baťa Health House in Zlín which brought together health and social services on one site. By 1936 it included partnerships with associations like the Red Cross, the Masaryk League for Combatting Tuberculosis, local leagues concerned with the health of young people and mothers and babies, the Health Centre of the Baťa Works and the District Health Insurance fund.[77] The key success of the institution lay in the way it brought these interests together to get the sick worker into the health system at an early point, thus reducing chronic and recurring illness and bringing down costs for the company and insurance fund.[78]

Despite these initiatives, many municipalities only provided simple hospice-style care in their institutions along with some infectious disease beds—though these might not be segregated. Thus, in 1926 in Bendzin, Silesia, the Rockefeller surveyor, Dr George Bevier, visited the hospital which he found to be:

> ...an old institution and under the Russian regime was a sort of "poor law hospital". It has been remodelled to some extent, but is not really satisfactory even now. It has an average of 80 to 90 patients per day, supports a small laboratory and an X Ray... There were many old ladies who were apparently chronics and we were told that it was the only place for old people. However, all were bed cases.[79]

The social care functions of hospitals were very evident in small town Hungary in the early 1930s, the director of a hospital in Miskolc writing that:

> Due to the grave economic situation, disjointed or absent family background, the shortage of food and housing, the hospital today is a shelter for the poor. Especially when the rainy and cold season comes, masses try to get admitted into the hospital... considering the social environment...some 15-20% of the patients treated have no serious illness but we replace their missing home with hospitalisation to give them back the ability to work.[80]

Yet the generally poor quality of much of the provision meant local populations were often sceptical about hospitals, Dr Ryder of Bendzin observing 'that people in this district usually object to going to hospital as they still associate it with dying and prefer to die at home. They have to be educated to go to hospital.'[81]

New-build hospitals were significantly larger, some with more than a thousand beds, and plans were in place for major projects, like that in Prague in the later 1930s. This envisaged creating a new 4,000 bed hospital with 32 clinics spread across two main blocks and a shared central service building, to replace the existing Czech and German university hospitals and medical schools. The new complex, which shared much in common with the project for the Regional Hospital in Lille,[82] envisaged state of the art planning in skyscraper tower blocks connected by bridges. The final 'hospital city' would have a Czech facility with 2,400 beds and twenty-two clinics while the German side would consist of 1,200 beds and ten clinics supported by a substantial shared medical school. The building was not developed but instead a new hospital was created in the suburbs at Motol and began taking patients in 1943.[83]

Figure 4.3: Plan for new Hospital and Medical School, Prague, 1937

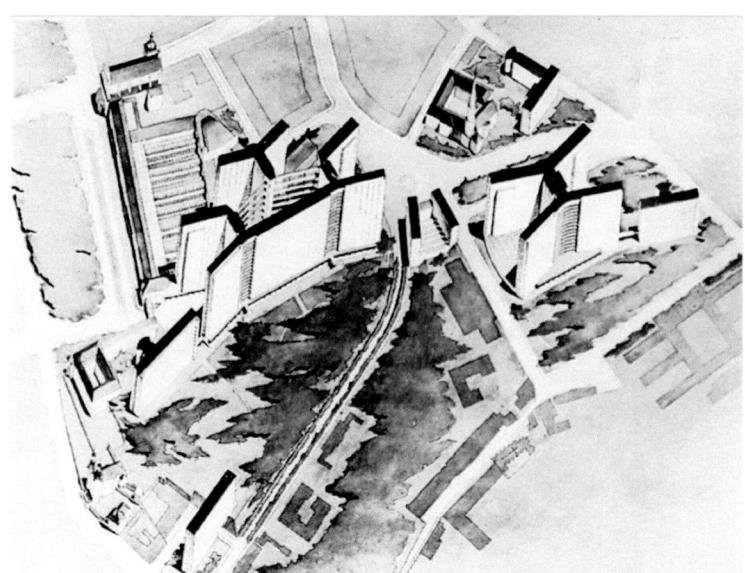

Source: J. Havlicek, V. Uklein, B. Albert, 'Study of A Health Centre and University Medical School at Prague', Nosokomeion, IX, 3 (1938), 210. (Reproduced with the permission of the Wellcome Collection)

This new building was underpinned by grandiose planning, including the district plans demanded by the Polish government in 1928 and the proposed Trapl-Albert plan in Czechoslovakia. The latter plan, produced by two medical doctors, Jiří Trapl and Bohuslav Albert, was published in 1933. Drawing on the experience at Zlín and US ideas about hierarchical regionalism, it proposed a merger of smaller uneconomical hospitals with larger provincial ones including the provision of social care and advice all in one institution or at least a set of affiliated institutions run from the centre. It had much in common with the health centre model promoted by Thomas Gruska with its focus on outpatient work as the primary function of institutional provision.[84] The plan formed the basis of a hospital bill introduced into the Czechoslovak parliament in 1937 but as a result of the worsening political situation this was shelved and not revived in the changed world of 1945.[85]

In all three countries nursing was in the hands of religious organisations. This was particularly the case in Poland, the most devoutly Roman Catholic of the three nations, but replacing the religious carers was a substantial task. There were few trained lay nurses and training facilities were limited. In 1922, Selskar Gunn found that in Poland nursing was largely 'done by nuns and on account of a strong catholic feeling it is difficult to dislodge them' while the country's leading health reformer, Ludwik Rajchman, thought them the 'most poisonous feature' of the Polish hospital situation.[86] It proved difficult for lay nurses to get training in hospitals dominated by nuns while 'the attitude of the medical profession towards the trained nurses is the same as that found in other continental countries, and it will take time to educate the doctors to the status of the trained nurses.'[87] In the 1920s Rockefeller's Elizabeth Crowell toured central Europe to establish the scale of training facilities—and the problem with untrained nurses—and built lasting networks to establish new schools.[88] However, Crowell and the RF generally favoured the training of public health nurses rather than the bedside staff the hospitals desperately required.[89] Moreover, neither hospitals nor doctors particularly wanted to see the nuns replaced. They were cheap, compliant and dedicated to care—essential for institutions which still dealt largely with the sick, infirm and chronic.[90] Nevertheless, by the late 1930s lay nurses dominated the hospitals of Budapest where the city's eleven public hospitals employed over 1000 nurses only 200 of which came from religious orders.[91]

Overall, the hospital services of these three nations were in the hands of multiple providers, with local authorities at the centre. The role of the central state was limited and outside of the big cities institutional care was largely in the hands of cash strapped counties and districts who concentrated on meeting the needs of the poorest. Non-state providers played a prominent role in Catholic Poland while employers managed a range of institutions in the industrial west.

Finance

As with provision, a mixed economy of finance existed across central Europe drawing on national insurance schemes, local taxes, state subsidies and private philanthropy as well as obligations imposed by government on employers. As noted, the former German, Austrian and Hungarian areas all inherited national insurance schemes from the former imperial systems but in the Russian territories no state scheme had been instituted before 1914. The benefits from these schemes were generous—certainly in terms of domiciliary and ambulatory services— and included some institutional care. Much of the responsibility for maintaining and treating hospital patients should have fallen to these schemes which were extended during the 1920s. But in each country the proportion of the population covered was low—usually less than 20 per cent. In particular, agricultural workers and peasant proprietors were excluded in all three countries, a major issue when up to three quarters of the population were involved in agriculture.[92] Hospital treatment was seen as expensive—a drain on the insurance funds' reserves— and an uncertain method of treatment. Strict conditions were applied. There was a requirement that institutional treatment would result in a cure, chronic diseases were excluded and benefit was usually time limited to four weeks—while domiciliary treatment could last up to a year. On the other hand, dependents were eligible for hospital treatment in both Hungary and Czechoslovakia.[93]

The widest scheme was in Czechoslovakia where a programme inherited from Austria was revised and extended on four occasions. It covered all workers with a contract and by 1938 around 3 million workers were included in the scheme, approximately 20% of the population.[94] Contributions were collected from employees and employers in equal proportions and administered by sickness funds overseen by a central social insurance institution and ultimately the Ministry of Social Welfare. The Key benefits were sickness benefit paid for up to a year—including dependents—GP ambulatory and domiciliary care, dentistry, access to a sick fund dispensary and some specialist treatment. Hospital treatment was available on a discretionary basis to cover maintenance and treatment in the lowest class of public hospital ward for up to four weeks. Further treatment beyond four weeks and admission for family members was optional to the fund. Tuberculosis sanatorium treatment could also be recommended where it was felt invalidity might be prevented. All hospital referrals were strictly controlled with GP recommendations approved by the Medical Officer of the Sickness Fund.

> 'The guiding principle laid down by the [Central Social Insurance] Institution make a distinction between cases in which hospital treatment is indispensible and those in which it is indicated by the presence of special conditions; they also enumerate the cases in which hospital treatment is not indicated.'[95]

Patients had to be admitted in the case of acute attacks, infectious diseases and where immediate surgical treatment was required. Ambiguous cases included those where: no specialist was available locally; housing conditions prevented effective treatment at home; the patient was too far from the GP for regular attendance; specialist diagnosis or treatment was required; a 'patient is recalcitrant to medical or other supervision'. But the GP and the Fund MO also had to ensure that admission was neither 'unduly prolonged' nor ended prematurely, 'negating the effects of treatment'. Exclusions encompassed chronic patients without the prospect of 'substantial improvement'; those who could be treated at home; and 'in particular, patients disabled by an incurable disease'.[96]

The social insurance scheme in Hungary was similar to Czechoslovakia, though it was more restrictive in terms of coverage with the focus on trade and industry, mining and state employees. The self-employed, including peasants, were therefore excluded. Access to benefits was also similar and included dependents who could be eligible for hospital treatment for up to four weeks. As with other schemes the focus was on a GP service closely regulated by the funds with some urban dispensaries, access to specialists including gynaecologists for home births and the whole overseen locally by a District Practitioner. There was significant central state control, with GPs employed on salary and the schemes regulated by statute.

Poland was the most complex as it necessitated the development of a new scheme to cover the whole nation. Although the Austrian system was the preferred model, it proved too expensive to contemplate and instead a watered-down version was rolled out across the nation in 1934. Insurance was compulsory for all wage earners with a contract and for salaried employees up to a certain level. Again, the self-employed, including tenant farmers and peasants, were excluded. Treatment was only available for 26 weeks, while dependents were eligible for just thirteen weeks' cover. In addition to GP, dental and specialist services, funds could grant free maintenance and treatment in the general class ward of a public hospital. As elsewhere, institutional treatment was reserved for those who could not be treated at home, the infectious, those who needed constant observation, and those who would not comply. Unlike the other schemes, there was a small co-payment element 'intended rather as a means of preventing unnecessary consultations than as a participation of the insured person in the cost of treatment.'[97]

Given the low coverage of the health insurance systems—especially in rural areas—the hospitals remained dependent on traditional sources of income to cover the cost of poor patients, though they were also able to open their doors to paying patients. The poorest patients were charged to the local authorities in Austrian areas or the central state through the counties in Hungarian regions. As in France this proved highly problematic in the era of rampant inflation that undermined the economies of Poland and Hungary until the late 1920s.[98] Municipal allocations—and even insurance payments - were frequently insufficient, either because the flat rate subvention did not cover the cost of patient treatment or because inflation ate into the daily rates paid. Thus, in industrial western Poland in the mid-1920s both midwives and doctors complained that the health insurance fund (the Kasa Chorych) 'pays not only poorly but very slowly'.[99] Even before the depression, Kasa Chorych was failing to meet its obligations, owing the hospitals of Warsaw almost two million zlotys in October 1929.[100] As the depression of the early 1930s peaked across Poland and Hungary, health insurance funds failed to pay to the hospitals and with a rising number of debtors, hospitals had to close wards and limit capacity. In Hungary, this was caused primarily by a shift in the means of paying for municipal patients. Up until 1930 the local authorities had paid a daily treatment rate but after this point a flat rate fee per capita was paid irrespective of the cost of the patient. Hospital managers calculated this was equivalent to a 50% reduction in the tariff while the number of indigent patients increased by around 20% to two thirds of all admissions due to the impact of the depression. One hospital director complained that 'Management by this fixed flat-rate is possible only in one of two ways. First, which the hospital has done, is to reduce the number of beds according to the state flat-rate; Second is to compromise the level of the treatment. Both of these are anti-social actions' but clearly ones being practiced by managers across the country.[101]

In one Hungarian hospital the number of debtors increased from sixteen in 1929 to 445 in 1936, around half of whom were insured patients and the rest poor patients who were the responsibility of the council.[102] More generally by 1932, Hungarian hospitals were operating at only 78% of capacity and one institution reported that it could only open 200 of its 600 beds due to lack of funds.[103] Although the situation in Czechoslovakia was less serious, the sharp increase in unemployment—to around one third of the insured population in 1933—meant the income of the schemes was substantially reduced. As a result the insured were forced back on to municipal support—also constrained by the depression—or charitable initiatives promoted by the government.[104] For each of these nations, the main weakness in the system was the exclusion of peasants from the insurance scheme. In an echo of the feudal era, it was expected that Hungarian landowners would meet the health costs of their tenants and workers. As the depression put significant downward pressure on agricultural prices and incomes many landowners defaulted on this obligation, forcing their peasantry onto the local state just as income from taxes was falling.

Hospitals set fees based on three classes of patient. In the Hungarian situation, which was similar to that elsewhere, third-class patients paid little or nothing with their costs met equally by the community of residence and the Ministry of Public Welfare (also the case in Slovakia and Polish Galicia). The insured were paid by the insurance fund. First-class patients had a private room, second-class shared two to three bedroom wards. This mix of public and private patients was different to the case in England or France—though similar to the US and Germany—and may have helped to supplement the income of hospitals in the difficult years around 1932 when all institutional funders were struggling.[105] Thus, at one small public hospital in north-east Hungary one in six patients paid for their own treatment, mostly in the third-class public wards, while just over ten per cent were covered by the insurance schemes and two thirds by the local state.[106] But there was also concern that potential paying patients were taking advantage of the hospitals to secure free treatment: 'It cannot be the interest of the provider, nor of the doctors, that wealthy patients, misusing the conditions, get beds, food cheaper than hotel prices, and medical care for free, at the public's expense.'[107]

There was also some philanthropic and charitable income within the sector, along with a range of institutions funded partly or wholly by employers and mutual funds. The primary philanthropic providers were religious bodies and ethnic groups who managed much of the chronic care along with services for specific communities. There was also a prominent contribution from the Red Cross. Although the Rockefeller Foundation did not fund hospitals directly it was instrumental in supporting the capital development of services, especially for research and nurse training for example in Prague and Cracow.[108]

Hospitals for a new nation

The countries that emerged from the collapse of the central European empires after 1918 had to build both coherent social, ethnic and political nations and strong states with modern services from their diverse inheritances. For Poland, Czechoslovakia and Hungary this involved the development of social welfare, and particularly health, infrastructure that would distinguish the new nations and build national identity. New hospitals, extended health insurance schemes, and modern social care facilities were created as evidence of the commitment of the new states to their people. In particular, each nation demonstrated a desire to create a modern, democratic health care system that reflected the power and status of an independent nation, free to make its own choices. This was especially evident in Poland where a myth had developed that the Russians had suppressed their original and well-developed hospital system. Writing in Nosokomeion in the 1930s various Polish authors pointed to the Russian fear of the Polish hospital services that led to them being placed under the dependence of political administrators and to their suppression for 'exclusively political motives'.[109]

Thus these new states attempted to build their identity through their health care policies in a range of areas. Most importantly they sought a uniform and generous health insurance scheme and each attempted to establish this by the 1930s—though often with limited operational effectiveness.[110] They also tried to develop curative hospitals over the caring regimes that dominated in the institutions they had inherited—especially in rural areas. The medical profession attempted to establish themselves as modern and progressive, even ahead of the traditional nations of Europe. In particular through the pages of *Nosokomeion*, they promoted the importance of the health centre model and of hospital led extra-mural services, with a Polish doctor active in public health management stating in 1934 that the 'modern hospital cannot longer be confined to its conventional work; it must dive into the masses and for that purpose it must go beyond its walls.'[111] They also sought to deliver uniform provision across the country both in terms of standard and quality of service and of management and administration. But this proved difficult given the persistence of different administrative systems for the delivery of hospital services in both Czechoslovakia and Poland.

Across the region, we see a focus on the name of the national leader—Masaryk in Czechoslovakia, Horthy in Hungary—and of symbolic national characters, like St Elizabeth. This naming process was particularly applied to new or controversial types of facility, like the Masaryk Homes development in Prague which saw traditional sick houses replaced by new social care facilities.[112] Similarly, in PKR the Czechoslovak state attempted to integrate the new region by improving health facilities—but with a nation building intent. The state had nationalised some of the region's hospitals and focused surpluses from the national insurance scheme on rebuilding projects in the east. Thus, the planned reconstruction of Ruthenia's Berehovo Provincial Hospital included a new maternity unit and a four-storey surgical block for male and female patients. Plans were also in place for three other new pavilions for internal, Ear, Nose and Throat, isolation and VD and skin.[113]

In Hungary, the new medical schools and hospitals were a defiant response to the losses suffered as a result of the treaty of Trianon. In the immediate pre-war period there had been a spate of new public hospitals (seven between 1900-1914) named Erzsébet after the national hero St Elizabeth of Hungary. However, a number of the new hospitals built in the 1920s and 1930s in border areas to replace institutions seceded to neighbours carried highly nationalistic names. The new institution for Bihar county on the Romanian border was named Count István Tisza, the prime minister of Hungary during the First World War who was assassinated at the beginning of the 'Aster Revolution' in October 1918. In Debrecen, where a new medical school was established, the hospital was called the Miklós Horthy Royal State Public Hospital while that in Szikszó took the name Ferenc II Rákóczi after the leader of a failed nationalist uprising of the early eighteenth century. There were at least two other Miklós Horthy hospitals, including an existing institution renamed after 1918.[114]

Further efforts to modernise and nationalise saw attempts to transform hospital personnel, replacing untrained nuns and patient helpers by nursing staff who had completed lengthy, accredited courses. They sought to ease out German, Austrian and Hungarian medical staff (there were still many German doctors in Silesia in the late 1920s),[115] while establishing skill and authority through schemes like the Rockefeller Fellowships and the

Figure 4.4: Plans for Berehovo Provincial Hospital, Ruthenia, 1933

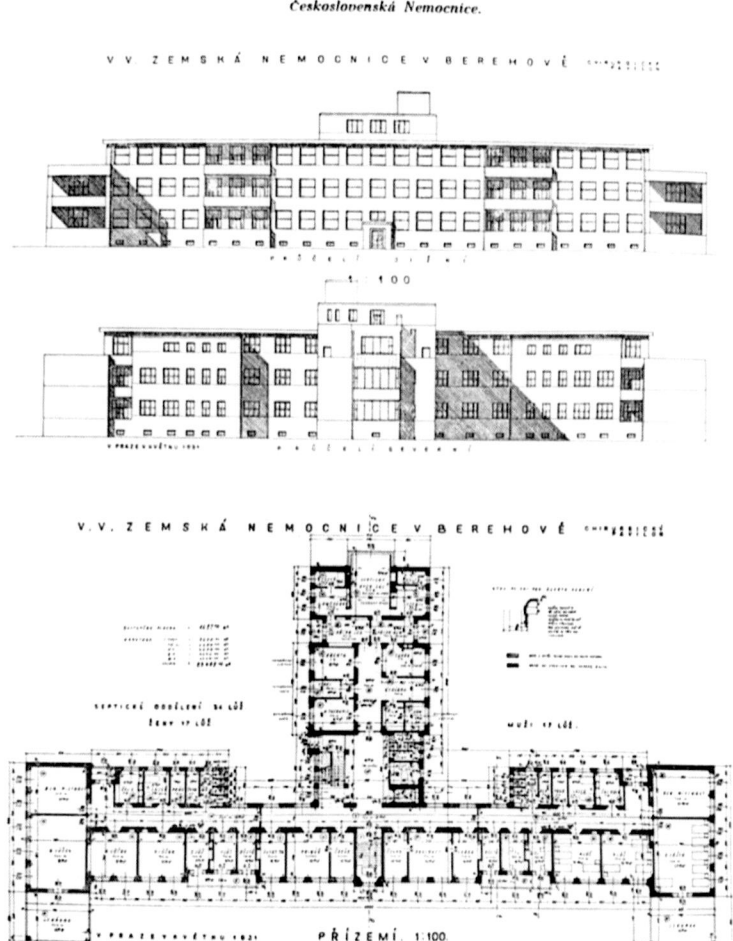

Source: Československá nemocnice, 3,5, 1933, 109 (Reproduced with the permission of the National Library of the Czech Republic)

establishment of national associations. They drew on western examples, and, where available, western advice and money.[116]

However, ethnic diversity made the creation of a unified health care system nearly impossible. Many cities had two or three large ethnic groups who often set up institutions to provide for their own. Duplication of services remained a severe problem, especially in elite institutions like universities, medical schools and even hospitals. For example, in Czechoslovakia, the German population maintained a prominent role in health provision and as a result both Czech and German speaking doctors were trained and practiced in Prague's main hospital, alternating clinics on a weekly basis. As the Czechs gradually took over Charles University, the Germans formed their own German University and Medical School. Thus when plans were developed for a new hospital in Prague city centre in the late 1930s, two separate buildings were envisaged with a 2,800 bed Czech institution and a 1,200 bed German facility on the same site sharing key services like catering, laundry and laboratories.[117] Jewish populations of the east also established a range of institutions for their own use. In the early 1920s separate nurse training schools existed for Jewish women, Gunn noting that 'in general it may be stated that the mixing of Jewish and gentile pupil nurses in the same school presents great difficulties' and he reported that a separate system for Jewish nurses was planned with schools in Warsaw, Łódź and Wilno where there were large Jewish hospitals to facilitate training.[118] As political tensions mounted at the end of the period the Rockefeller Foundation found that the Germans refused to share a new nurse training institution they were willing to fund and insisted on their own classes in German. They eventually walked out and formed their own school in 1938.[119]

The experience of these three states is paradigmatic of the experience of most of the post-imperial nations of interwar Central and South-East Europe formed by the break-up of the four empires.

These were largely multi-ethnic nations that drew on two or more imperial inheritances. Economically they were rural and as such struggled to raise the levels of finance needed for a modern health care system—a task made more difficult by rampant inflation in the 1920s and by the Great Depression in the early 1930s. But their inheritances also meant they could benefit from the existence of well-established national insurance schemes and a basic hospital infrastructure with professional staff trained mostly in the German/Austrian system. The central states were also determined to modernise and extend the system—with some success. Certainly, by 1938 the number and quality of hospital beds had expanded, with concerted attempts to improve provision in the least developed areas of eastern Poland and Czechoslovakia and in central Hungary. The later 1930s saw each nation, and especially Hungary, launch extensive schemes to extend access to and provision of hospitals, while specialist, and especially maternity services, became more widespread. But delivering this proved to be a significant challenge as economic crisis, political instability and ethnic conflict undermined these schemes, while the rural nature of these countries limited their ability to create a robust health infrastructure. Moreover, the ambition to create unified and universal systems proved very difficult to fulfil, particularly in Czechoslovakia where political and ethnic conflict saw the country become less integrated by the end of the period. The ambition of these countries to create inclusive, modern health care for the new nation foundered on the central state's inability to fund, or create the environment for, a uniform model while the contribution of non-state actors proved patchy and parochial. Yet overall, the interwar period did see these countries improve their hospital services significantly and position health as a major political feature of their political ambitions.

1. We would like to thank the University of Huddersfield's University Research Fund for supporting this research and the Rockefeller Archive Centre for their generous Research Stipend Award which allowed me to complete research in the Rockefeller Foundation collection. Translations from Polish are by Melissa Hibbard, from Czech by Frank Grombir and from Hungarian by Balázs Szélinger.

2. Steven Cherry, Medical Services and the Hospitals in Britain, 1860-1939 (Cambridge: Cambridge University Press, 1996); Martin Gorsky, John Mohan and Martin Powell, 'The Financial Health of Voluntary Hospitals in Interwar Britain', Economic History Review, 55 (2002), 533-57; Barry M. Doyle, The Politics of Hospital Provision in Early Twentieth Century Britain (London: Pickering and Chatto, 2014); George C. Gosling, Payment and Philanthropy in British Healthcare, 1918-48 (Manchester: Manchester University Press, 2017).

3. J.P. Domin, Une histoire economique de l'hôpital, XIXe-XXe siècles: Une analyse rétrospective du développement hospitalier, 2 vols. (Paris: La Documentation Française, 2008); Timothy B Smith, 'The Social Transformation of Hospitals and the Rise of Medical Insurance in France, 1914-1943', Historical Journal 41, 4 (1998), 1055-87; Margarita Vilar-Rodriguez and Jerònia Pons-Pons, 'Competition and collaboration between public and private sectors: the historical construction of the Spanish hospital system, 1942–86', Economic History Review, 72, 4 (2019), 1384-1408; E.P. Hennock, The Origin of the Welfare State in England and Germany, 1850–1914: Social Policies Compared (Cambridge: Cambridge University Press, 2007). See also Axel Hüntelmann & Oliver Falk (eds) Accounting for Health: Calculative Practices and Administrative Techniques, 1500-2000 (Manchester, Manchester University Press, forthcoming 2021) and Marius Turda 'Private and public traditions of healthcare in Central and South-eastern Europe, from the nineteenth to the (mid-) twentieth centuries', in Paul Weindling (ed), Healthcare in Private and Public from the Early Modern Period to 2000 (London: Routledge, 2015), 101-122.

4. For example, Richard Freeman, The Politics of Health in Europe (Manchester: Manchester University Press, 2000), 14-23.

5. Martin Gorsky, John Mohan and Martin Powell, 'British Voluntary Hospitals, 1871-1938: The Geography of Provision and Utilization', Journal of Historical Geography 25 (1999), 463-482; Alysa Levene, Martin Powell, John Stewart and Becky Taylor, Cradle to Grave: Municipal Medicine in Interwar England and Wales (Bern: Peter Lang, 2011); Barry M Doyle, 'Les soins hospitaliers en Grande-Bretagne pendant l'entre-deux-guerres: un marché de la santé ?', in Bruno Valat (ed.), Marches de la sante en Europe au XXe siècle (Toulouse: Presses Universitaires du Midi, 2020); Barry M. Doyle, 'Healthcare before welfare states: Hospitals in early twentieth century England and France', Canadian Bulletin of Medical History, 33 (2016), 174-204; Vilar-Rodriguez and Pons-Pons, op. cit. (note 3).

6. Martin Gorsky, John Mohan with Tim Willis, Mutualism and Health Care: British Hospital Contributory Schemes in the Twentieth Century (Manchester: Manchester University Press, 2006); Timothy B. Smith, Creating the Welfare State in France, 1880-

1940 (Montreal: McGill-Queen's University Press, 2003); Doyle, 'Healthcare', op. cit., (note 5); Hennock, op. cit., (note.3).

7. International Labour Office (ILO), Economical Administration of Health Insurance Benefits (Geneva: ILO, 1938).

8. Frank Grombir, Melissa Hibbard, Balázs Szélinger and Barry M. Doyle, 'Hospital Provision in Interwar Central Europe: A Review of the Field', European Review of History (forthcoming 2021).

9. Petr Svobodný, Helena Hnilicová, Hana Janečková, Eva Křížová, Hana Mášová, 'Continuity and Discontinuity of Health and Health Care in the Czech Lands during two Centuries (1800-2000)', Hygiea Internationalis, 4, 1 (2004), 81-107; Hana Mášová, 'Czechoslovak hospital reform in the 1930s', in Martin Dinges (ed.), Health and Health Care between Self-Help, Intermediary Organizations and Formal Poor Relief, 1500-2005 (Lisboa: Edições Colibri, 2007), 169-182; Hana Mášová and Petr Svobodný, 'Health and health care in Czechoslovakia 1918-1938: From infectious to civilisation diseases', in Iris Borowy and W.D. Gruner (eds), Facing Illness in Troubled Times: Health in Europe in the Interwar Years 1918-1939 (Oxford: Peter Lang, 2005), 165-205; Hana Mášová, Nemocniční otázka v meziválečném Československu (Prague: Karolinum, 2005).

10. M. Godycki-Ćwirko, M. Oleszczyk, A. Windak, 'The Development of Primary Health Care in Poland from the 2nd Republic to the Round Table Agreement (1918–1989)', Problemy Medycyny Rodzinnej, 12 (2010) 29-36.

11. Though see Tomasz Inglot, Welfare States in East Central Europe, 1919-2004 (New York: Cambridge University Press, 2008); Bela Tomka, Welfare in East and West. Hungarian Social Security in an International Comparison, 1918-1990 (Berlin: Akademie Verlag, 2004).

12. Karel Černý, 'History of medicine in the Czech Republic: past and present', Istoriya meditsiny, 3, 2 (2016), 190-193.

13. Paul Weindling, Epidemics and Genocide in Eastern Europe, 1890–1945 (Oxford: Oxford University Press, 2000); Marius Turda, Eugenics and Nation in Early 20th Century Hungary (Basingstoke: Palgrave Macmillan, 2014); Erik Ingebrigtsen, 'Privileged origins: "national models" and reforms of public health in interwar Hungary', Györgi Peteri (ed.) Imagining the West in Eastern Europe and the Soviet Union (Pittsburgh: University of Pittsburgh Press, 2010).

14. John Farley, To Cast Out Disease: A History of the International Health Division of the Rockefeller Foundation (1913–1951) (New York and Oxford: Oxford University Press, 2004).

15. Ilana Löwy and Patrick Zylberman, 'Introduction: Medicine as a Social Instrument: Rockefeller Foundation, 1913–45', Studies in the History and Philosophy of Biology & Biomedical Science, 31, 3 (2000), 365–379 and contributions to the Special Issue by Marta Aleksandra Balinska, 'The Rockefeller Foundation and the National Institute of Hygiene, Poland, 1918–45', 419-432 and Gábor Palló 'Rescue and Cordon Sanitaire: The Rockefeller Foundation in Hungarian Public Health', 433-445; Paul Weindling, 'Public Health and Political Stabilisation: The Rockefeller Foundation in Central and

Eastern Europe Between The Two World Wars', Minerva, 31 (1993), 253-267; Benjamin B. Page, 'The Rockefeller Foundation and Central Europe: A Reconsideration', Minerva, 40 (2002), 265-87.

16. For a discussion of the use of welfare more generally as a nation building tool in central Europe after 1918 see Inglot, op. cit. (note 11).

17. Grombir et al, op. cit. (note 8).

18. Jiří Říha (ed.), Zdravotnická ročenka Československa 1928-1940, (Vols. I-XI), (Praha: Piras 1928-40).

19. Ministerstwo Opieki Społecznej, Dwadzieścia lat publicznej służby zdrowia w Polsce odrodzonej, 1918-1938 (Warsaw: Nakładem Ministerstwa Opieki Społecznej, 1939).

20. League of Nations (LoN), International Health Yearbook 1924-30 (Vol. I-VI) (Geneva: League of Nations, 1925-32); ILO, op. cit. (note 7).

21. Farley, op. cit. (note 14).

22. Robert Bideleux, A History of Eastern Europe: Crisis and Change, 2nd edn (London: Routledge, 2007).

23. Ian Kershaw, To Hell and Back: Europe, 1914-1949 (London: Penguin, 2016), 114-21.

24. Cynthia Paces, 'Public Health Networks, Eugenics, and the Birth of Czechoslovakia', European Review of History (Forthcoming, 2021).

25. Inglot, op. cit. (note 11). For a similar situation in Ireland see Donnacha Séan Lucey, The End of the Irish Poor Law: Welfare and Healthcare Reform in Revolutionary and Independent Ireland (Manchester: Manchester University Press, 2015).

26. Tomka, op. cit. (note 11).

27. Anita J. Prażmowska, A History of Poland, 2nd edn (Basingstoke: Palgrave, 2011).

28. Mary Heimann, Czechoslovakia: The State that Failed (New Haven Ct.: Yale University Press, 2011).

29. Miklós Molnár, A Concise History of Hungary (Cambridge: Cambridge University Press, 2001).

30. Petr Svobodný and Ludmila Hlaváčková, Dějiny lékařství v českých zemích [The history of medicine in the Czech Lands] (Triton, Praha: 2004); Ludmila Hlaváčková; Petr Svobodný; Jan Bříza, History of the General University Hospital in Prague (Prague: Všeobecná fakultní nemocnice v Praze, 2014).

31. Nadav Davidovitch and Rakefet Zalashik, '"Air, sun, water": Ideology and activities of OZE (Society for the preservation of the health of the Jewish population) during the interwar period', Dynamis, 28 (2008), 127-149.

32. Rockefeller Archive Center (RAC) RG6/ SG1/395/45/523, Selskar M. Gunn, 'Public Health in Hungary, September 1924'; RAC RG6/SG1/395/47/528, Selskar M. Gunn, 'Report on Poland, 1922'; RAC RG6/ SG1/395/49/546, Wickliffe Rose and S.M. Gunn, 'Public Health in Czechoslovakia, 1921'; Cynthia Paces, 'Eugenics and Public Health: the Birth of the Czechoslovak State',

33. Prażmowska, op. cit. (note 26).

34. RAC RG6/SG1/395/47/528, Gunn, op. cit. (note 31), 31-36 and Appendix, 3.

35. RAC RG6/SG1/395/45/523, Gunn, op. cit. (note 31), Appendix F.

36. I.T. Berend and G Ránki, Economic Development in East-Central Europe in the 19th and 20th Centuries (New York: Columbia University Press, 1974), 214-223.

37. RAC RG6/SG1/395/45/523, Gunn, op. cit. (note 31); RAC RG6/SG1/395/47/528, Gunn, op. cit. (note 31); RAC RG6/SG1/395/49/546, Rose and Gunn, op. cit. (note 31); Inglot, op. cit. (note 11), ch.2. But for a less rosy assessment of Czechoslovakia see Heimann, op. cit. (note 27) and Page, op. cit. (note 15).

38. Grombir et al, op. cit. (note 8).

39. RAC, Officers' diaries, RG 12, S-Z (FA394), G.K Strode Diary 24 September 1927. See also RAC RG1.1/712J/386/5/48 Medzilaborce Public Health Survey, 1930-32; RAC RG1.1/712J/386/5/50 Turciansky Svaty Martin Health Demonstration, 1926-30 for RF work in Slovakia in the 1920s; Frank Grombir, 'Mission impossible? The hospital provision in Subcarpathian Ruthenia, Czechoslovakia's easternmost province, 1918-1938', Unpublished paper, European Association for the History of Medicine and Health Conference, Bucharest, 2017.

40. Inglot, op. cit. (note 11), ch.2.

41. RAC RG1.1/712J/386/5/48, op. cit. (note 38).

42. E.A. Valchuk, 'Medical and Sanitary Practice in Lida County (Nowogródek Province) at the Time of the Second Rzeczpospolita (1919-1939)', Archiwum Historii i Filozofii Medycyny 77 (2014), 9-15.

43. Turda op. cit. (note 3), 113.

44. LoN, International Health Yearbook 1930 (Vol.VI), op. cit. (note 19), 'Czechoslovakia', 101-136 at 121-23; 'Hungary', 397-432 at 419. LoN, International Health Yearbook 1929 (Vol. V), op. cit. (note 19), 'Poland', 869-70.

45. RAC RG6/SG1/395/45/523, Gunn, op. cit. (note 31); RAC RG6/SG1/395/47/528, Gunn, op. cit. (note 31); RAC RG6/SG1/395/49/546, Rose and Gunn, op. cit. (note 31).

46. Václav Veselý, 'Státní epidemické autokolony', Zdravotnická ročenka Československa, IV (1931), 52–53.

47. On Czechoslovakia, Theodor Gruschka, 'The Hospital as a Centre of the Health Work in the District', Nosokomeion, IV,2 (1933), 264-5; on Poland, T. Mogilnicki, 'Le role social du medecin de l'hopital rural', Nosokomeion V,1 (1934), 47–51. See also the health demonstration work in Czechoslovakia in note 39.

48. Tomka, op.cit. (note 11), 128 and 134; Inglot, op.cit. (note 11), ch.2.

49. For more detail on these different systems see below.

50. See Barry Doyle, 'What's in a Name? What is a Hospital? Part 2' https://healthcarebeforewelfarestates.wordpress.com/2017/08/11/what-is-a-hospital-part-2-whats-in-a-name/ [accessed 13.01.2019]

51. See the discussions of Britain and France in George Weisz, Chronic Disease in the Twentieth Century: A History (Baltimore: Johns Hopkins University Press, 2014).

52. Mental hospitals, infectious diseases and even chronic care are often excluded from the hospital historiography of Britain. See the works in notes 2 and 5 above. John V. Pickstone, Medicine and Industrial Society: A History of Hospital Development in Manchester and Its Region (Manchester: Manchester University Press, 1985) is good on provision for all types of physical complaints. For a regional study of mental health provision in the early twentieth century see Alice Brumby, 'From 'Pauper Lunatics' to 'Rate-Aided Patients': Dismantling the Poor Law of Lunacy in Mental Health Care: 1888-1930' (unpublished PhD thesis: University of Huddersfield, 2015).

53. Brian Abel-Smith, The Hospitals, 1800-1948: A Study in Social Administration in England and Wales (London: Publisher missing 1964); Christian Chevandier, L'Hôpital dans la France du XXe Siècle (Paris: Perrin, 2009); Rosemary Stevens, In Sickness and in Wealth: American Hospitals in the Twentieth Century, (New York: Basic Books, 1989).

54. This is explored by Lucey, op. cit. (note 24).

55. Witold Przywieczerski, 'Les Hopitaux en Pologne', Nosokomeion, V, 1 (1934), 140-143.

56. Ministerstwo Opieki Społecznej, op. cit. (note 18), 97.

57. Zdravotnická ročenka Československa, op. cit. (note 18).

58. Magyarország gyógyintézeteinek évkönyve, op.cit. (note 18); RAC RG1.1/750C/386/2/22 'Debrecen School of Nursing, 1925-1933, 1936'.

59. Przywieczerski, op. cit. (note 54), 141.

60. Hynek Pelc, Organisation of the Public Health Services in Czechoslovakia (Geneva: League of Nations, 1925). Grombir, op. cit. (note 38)

61. Grombir, op. cit. (note 38).

62. RAC RG6/SG1/395/45/523, Gunn, op. cit. (note 31), 158.

63. Grombir, et al, op. cit. (note 8); RAC RG1.1/750A/386/2/11-12, 'University of Szeged'.

64. For the situation in the US, England and France see Stevens, op. cit. (note 52); Doyle, 'Healthcare', op. cit. (note 5).

65. RAC RG6/SG1/395/45/523, Gunn, op. cit. (note 31), 153.

66. Ibid.; I. Dobrossy, 'Miskolc infrastruktúrájának modernizálása és a Speyer Bank-

kölcsön felhasználása', in A. Herman (ed.) A Hermann Ottó Múzeum Évkönyve. (Miskolc: Herman Ottó Múzeum, 1996), 423-450. The loans from the US Speyer Bank, formed part of a League of Nations sponsored financial restructuring of Hungary in the mid-1920s which focused on lending to improve industrial and state infrastructure. Tamás Magyarics, 'Balancing in Central Europe: Great Britain and Hungary in the 1920s', in Aliaksandr Piahanau (ed.), Great Power Policies towards Central Europe, 1914-1945, (E-IR Publishing) https://www.e-ir.info/2019/03/13/balancing-in-central-europe-great-britain-and-hungary-in-the-1920s/.

67. Following post-war hyper-inflation in Hungary that made the korona effectively worthless, the Pengő was introduced in 1927 as part of the economic restructuring promoted by the League of Nations. It proved relatively successful in stabilising the economy and trade and controlling inflation until the Second World War.

68. Zoltán Takács, 'Horthy Miklós Városi Közhórház, Nagykanizsa', Magyar Kórház, Supplement to Vol. V (1936) 'Register of Hungarian Healthcare Institutions', 247-62. See also Emil Wallner, 'Veszprém megyei város közkórháza', Magyar Kórház, Supplement to Vol. V (1936) 'Register of Hungarian Healthcare Institutions', 263-78 for extensions funded by Speyer loan, 1930-33.

69. Maciek Godycki-Ćwirko, Marek Oleszczyk, and Adam Windak, 'The Development of Primary Health Care in Poland from the 2nd Republic to the Round Table Agreement (1918–1989)', Lekarz rodzinny, XII, 1 (2010), 29-36.

70. S.B Walsh, Handbook of Employees Service Social Insurance Giesche Spółka Akcyjna (P.P. 1928)

71. Ministerstwo Opieki Społecznej, op. cit. (note 18), 96.

72. Magdalena Grassmann, Agnieszka Zemke-Górecka and Kędra Bogusław. 'Szpitalnictwo cywilne w województwie białostockim w II Rzeczpospolitej'Miscellanea Historico-Iuridica, 8 (2009), 141-2.

73. Przywieczerski, op. cit. (note 54), 141; Veselý, op. cit. (note 45).

74. RAC RG6/SG1/395/47/528, Gunn, op. cit. (note 31), 11.

75. Przywieczerski, op. cit. (note 54), 142.

76. Ibid., 136. This contrasts with England and the US where private hospitals resisted merger or closure. Barry M. Doyle 'Competition and Cooperation in Hospital Provision in Middlesbrough, 1918-48', Medical History, 51 (2007), 337-56; Stevens, op. cit. (note 52).

77. Vlad. Uklein, B. Albert, D. Tolar, 'Das Bata-Haus Der Gesundheit in Zlin', Nosokomeion, VII, 2 (1936), 128-39.

78. Uklein, Albert and Tolar, op. cit. (note 77).

79. RAC RG1.1/789J/386/4/50, 'Poland, Health Demonstrations: Bendzin Report, 1926. Memorandum of Visit to Bendzin, Poland, Bevier, November 7-8, 1925', 12-13.

80. Gyula Jäger, 'Szociális takarékosság a racionalizált közkórházban', Magyar Kórház, Supplement to Vol. IV 1 (1935) 'Register of

Hungarian Healthcare Institutions', 7.

81. RAC RG1.1/789J/386/4/50, 'Poland, Health Demonstrations: Bendzin Report, 1926, op.cit. (note 79), 15.

82. https://bmdoyleblog.wordpress.com/2014/02/06/pie-in-the-sky-paul-nelsons-design-for-the-cite-hospitaliere-de-lille-1932/ [accessed 2.2.2019]; Julie Willis, Philip Goad and Cameron Logan, Architecture and the Modern Hospital: Nosokomeion to Hygeia (London: Routledge, 2019), 188-202.

83. J. Havlicek, V. Uklein, D. Albert, 'Study of A Health Centre and University Medical School at Prague', Nosokomeion, (1938), 202-221; Hlaváčková,Svobodný, Bříza, op. cit. (note 29).

84. See for example, Theodor Gruschka, 'Die Praventiven Aufgaben Des Krankenhauses', Nosokomeion, IV, 1 (1933), 6-13.

85. Masova, op. cit. (note 9).

86. RAC RG6/SG1/395/47/528, Gunn, op. cit. (note 31), 26.

87. RAC RG6/SG1/395/47/528, Gunn, op. cit. (note 31), 28.

88. Elizabeth D. Vickers, 'Frances Elizabeth Crowell and the politics of nursing in Czechoslovakia after the First World War', Nursing History Review, 7, 1 (1999), 67-96.

89. For reports by Frances Crowell on nursing in Poland see the files in RAC RG1.1/789c/386/3/29-32 especially 'Memorandum re: sick nursing and health visiting, 1922' and 'University of Cracow: Public health and bedside nursing'.

90. For a similar situation in France see Katrin Schultheiss, Bodies and Souls: Politics and the Professionalization of Nursing in France, 1880–1922 (Cambridge, MA: Harvard University Press, 2001).

91. Béla Ródé, 'A székesfőváros közkórházainak deiglenes alkalmazottai', Magyar Kórház, Supplement 11, Vol. VI (1937) 'Register of Hungarian Healthcare Institutions', 207-14.

92. LoN, International Health Yearbook 1930, op. cit. (note 19), 101-136; 397-432; 677-718; ILO, op. cit. (note 7); Inglot, op. cit. (note 11).

93. ILO, op. cit. (note 7); Inglot, op. cit. (note 11).

94. LoN, op. cit. (note 19).

95. ILO, op. cit. (note 7), 156.

96. ILO, op. cit. (note 7), 47-56.

97. ILO, op. cit. (note 7), 234.

98. For the situation in France see Barry M. Doyle 'Contrasting accounting practices in the urban hospitals of England and France, 1890s to1930s', in Hüntelmann and Falk (eds), op. cit. (note 3).

99. RAC RG1.1/789J/386/4/50 Poland Health Demonstrations: Bendzin Report 1926, 11.

100. Zofia Podgórska-Klawe, Szpitale Warszawskie, 1388-1945, (Warsaw: Państwowe Wydawnictwo Naukowe, 1975), 292.

101. Jäger Gyula, 'Borsodvármegye Erzsébet közkórháza, Miskolc', Magyar Kórház, Supplement to Vol. IV (1935) 'Register of Hungarian Healthcare Institutions', 209-222.

102. Figures for Hódmezővásárhely Public Hospital, the Hódmezővásárhely Municipal Archives in Csongrád County (CSML-HL) CSML-HL VIII. 802. Vols 47-48.

103. Grombir et al, op. cit. (note 8).

104. Pavel Victor Ovseiko, 'The Politics of Health Care Reform in Central and Eastern Europe: The Case of the Czech Republic', (Unpublished D.Phil. thesis: University of Oxford, 2008), 64-7.

105. George C. Gosling, Payment and Philanthropy in British Healthcare, 1918-48 (Manchester: Manchester University Press, 2017); Olivier Faure and Dominique Dessertine, Les cliniques priveés: Deux siècles de success, (Rennes: Presses Universitaires de Rennes, 2012); Stevens, op. cit. (note 52); Hüntelmann in Hüntelmann and Falk, op. cit. (note 3).

106. Tóth Ernő: 'Abauj-Torna vármegye "II Rákóczi Ferenc" közkórháza, Szikszón', Magyar Kórház, 2, 4 (1933), 129-132.

107. Borszéky Károly: 'Időszerű kórházi problémák', Magyar Kórház, 1, 1 (1932), 10-14. For similar concerns in England see Doyle, 'marché de la santé', op. cit. (note 5).

108. Farley, op. cit. (note 14); RAC RG1.1/789C/386/3/33 'University of Cracow, Public Health Bedside Nursing, 1925-37'.

109. Przywieczerski, op. cit. (note 54); Boleslaw Jakimiak, 'La Legislation Polonaise Concernant les Hospitaux et son Development, Nosokomeion, 2 (1934), 106-119 at 110.

110. ILO, op. cit. (note 7).

111. T. Mogilnicki, 'Le role social du medecin de l'hopital rural', Nosokomeion, V, 1 (1934), 47-51.

112. Hana Mášová, 'O stavbě Masarykových domovů, sociálních ústavů hlavního města Prahy', Dějiny věd a techniky, 29, 2 (1996), 101-116.

113. Svatopluk Veselý, 'Rekonstrukce zemské nemocnice v Berehově', Československá nemocnice, 3,5, 1933, 107-10.

114. Magyarország gyógyintézeteinek évkönyve, op. cit. (note 18).

115. Walsh, op. cit. (note 69).

116. RAC RG1.1/789c/386/3/29-32, Reports by Frances Crowell on nursing in Poland,; Weindling, op. cit. (note 15); Page, op. cit. (note 15); RAC RG6/SG1/395/47/528, Gunn, op. cit. (note 31), 20-1.

117. Havlicek, Uklein and Albert, op. cit. (note 82), 207; Hlaváčková, Svobodný, Bříza, op. cit. (note 29).

118. RAC RG6/SG1/395/47/528, Gunn, op. cit. (note 31), 29.

119. RAC RG5/3-700115/243/2933, 'Annual Report for 1938, Paris Office, IHD. Section IV: Italy, Albania, Austria, Czechoslovakia, Hungary and Poland'.

Chapter 5

Public, private and voluntary hospitals: economic theory and historical experience in Britain, c.1800-2010

Martin Gorsky
(London School of Hygiene and Tropical Medicine)

Introduction

In considering the balance of public and private in the history of the British hospital, we may helpfully think in three, rather than just two categories: public, private and 'voluntary'. We may also distinguish different periods, particularly across the juncture of 1948, when the establishment of the National Health Service (NHS) disrupted existing patterns of ownership and financing and heralded a period of active management by the central state. Crudely we can classify the public hospitals as those funded principally by taxation and overseen by some appointed or elected body subject to statutory regulation. The private hospitals we may consider as those run for profit and privately owned. The voluntary hospitals we may understand as those financed principally by philanthropy or mutual funds, staffed largely by honorary consultants, constituted as charitable trusts and managed by volunteer committees. In the British narrative, the for-profit hospitals do not figure significantly, though there were numerous nursing and maternity homes, commercial 'lunatic asylums' and private beds or wings within voluntary hospitals; private hospitals remained of limited scale under the NHS. Thus, the dynamic of most interest is that between the voluntary and public sectors before 1948, and within the public sector afterwards.

The British hospital has an established narrative of change, broadly understood as a social response to industrialisation.[1] The public hospital emerged from the Poor Law workhouse and was systematically developed in the Victorian period. Psychiatric hospitals—'asylums'—were predominantly provided by county or municipal councils and from the 1870s local government also oversaw isolation hospitals for infectious diseases. Voluntary hospitals emerged in the eighteenth century, then proliferated, generally prioritising acute but non-infectious diseases, and leaving long-stay, 'chronic' and psychiatric patients to the public sector. This changed in the twentieth century as municipal hospitals and public infirmaries expanded general care. A radical break occurred in 1948, when the NHS Acts took the voluntary hospitals into public ownership, also incorporating local government hospitals, public asylums and many ex-Poor Law institutions. NHS history breaks into an early statist period marked by central planning, albeit ineffective, then from the 1980s an effort to introduce market disciplines under the aegis of 'neo-liberalism'. There was also a trend of dehospitalisation, as technological and surgical processes allowed for shorter stays and community treatment.

The aim of this chapter is to explain the changing relationship between public, private and voluntary sectors over this long period. As a framing device, it will use a body of theory drawn principally from welfare economics, which makes normative claims about the strengths and weaknesses of each sector. After introducing these ideas, the discussion that follows asks how adequately they address four questions that are not usually confronted explicitly:

1. How to explain the growth of the hospital since the eighteenth century, and the distribution of activity between private, public and voluntary sectors?
2. How to explain the transfer of control from the voluntary sector and local government to the central state in the NHS system reform of 1946-8?
3. How to explain the pattern of decline of the hospital in the later twentieth century, and the distribution of activity between the public and private sectors?
4. How to explain and appraise the market-oriented management reforms adopted in the NHS since the 1980s?

The analysis synthesises existing work based on what is already a rich literature, combining policy history with a strong quantitative underpinning.

Market, voluntary and state failure

A preliminary conceptual framework to aid thinking about the sectoral dynamics of the British hospital is presented in Figure 5.1. This proposes various positive 'virtues' of the market, voluntary institutions, and the state as providers of health care, and also various inherent 'failures' that may explain why each predominates at different times. As outlined below, it is constructed from the longstanding literature of welfare economists, and more recently from the fields of health economics and third sector analysis.

Figure 5.1: A conceptual model of hospital sectors in time

	Market	Voluntary	State
Virtues	Price mechanism; responsive to demand; quality.	Mobilises supply; resolves trust failures; innovation; advocacy.	Sufficiency of supply; resolves trust failures; integrated planning.
Failures	Free riders; information asymmetries; trust failures; insufficiency for catastrophic costs	Free riders; insufficiency; unevenness; paternalism; uncoordinated; amateurism.	Bureaucratic maximising; rent-seeking, 'provider capture'; no voice or exit.
Change	Transition from voluntary/local/private towards public.		
Change	'objective reasons of a stringent nature'; 'majority opinion'; changing 'social ideas'; 'displacement effects' of war.		

It is axiomatic to classical economic theory that free markets can most directly satisfy human needs. Competition drives innovation and quality, the price mechanism optimises the balance between supply and demand, and an 'invisible hand' ensures that by meeting individual utility markets will increase the general welfare.[2] However, theory had also to contend with the growth of public expenditure. Adolph Wagner's 'law', propounded in Bismarckian Germany, first claimed this as an inexorable concomitant of economic growth.[3] Later there developed the concept of public goods, whose benefits ('positive externalities') extended to all, not just their immediate purchasers—urban sanitation systems that reduce infectious disease, for example. To avert 'free riding' by other beneficiaries, collective intervention could be justified. Another market failure could arise from imperfect information, where the purchaser lacked the requisite knowledge to assess the price of a technically complex service, such as medicine. This introduced a 'trust failure', where sellers might be tempted to profiteer, particularly if, as in the case of doctors, they exercised a professional monopoly. It was also arguable that health care was not really a consumer good at all, because the catastrophic expense of serious illness might price supply beyond the means of average earners.[4]

What about voluntarism? An economic 'language of sectors' emerged in the mid-twentieth century, making general claims about the capabilities and limits of charity, as it reoriented under the welfare state.[5] This asserted the voluntary sector's role was to pioneer new forms of intervention, reach hitherto neglected groups, produce individualised services, and advocate for change. In this sense, it could address insufficiencies of supply when catastrophic costs threatened and, because it was premised on philanthropic ethics, could resolve trust failures. It was also unfettered by the bureaucracy or need for consent that accompanied state action.[6] However, voluntary failures were also observed. The problem remained of free riders enjoying the positive externalities funded by charitable citizens alone, not least in public health.[7] Other weaknesses were a lack of co-ordinating mechanisms, undemocratic governance, under-resourcing, amateurism of the workforce and political ineffectiveness. Third sector theorists subsequently augmented this catalogue. Philanthropy was inherently insufficient and geographically uneven, because its spontaneous nature, its reliance on wealthy givers, and its lack of coordinating mechanisms meant that supply could not match demand. Charity's paternalist and hierarchical overtones also offended equity considerations.[8]

These failures opened the way for the state. Whether through mandatory insurance or social security, public funding ensured sufficiency of supply while averting free riding in the provision of public goods. Planned distribution could overcome geographical or social unevenness, and bureaucrats appointed on merit could deliver professional administration. Trust failures from information asymmetries could be overcome through expert oversight of pricing, and sanctions. Yet against these virtues, the lineaments of state failure were soon set out, both by Hayekian neo-liberals and by rational choice theorists. Because bureaucrats seek to maximise their own utility rather than pursuing the public interest, they will try always to enlarge departmental budgets to obtain status and power.[9] Nor does the state necessarily prevent rent-seeking by professionals.[10] Instead there is a tendency to 'provider capture' by public employees—doctors, nurses, administrators—who organise services to suit their own preferences, not the consumers'.[11] The patient meanwhile lacked the levers of 'voice and exit', which in market settings would permit the expression of demand.[12]

So much for theory—what about application to historical examples? To the extent they exist, these addressed the supersession of voluntary, local or market approaches by the central state. Wagner had attributed his 'law' to technological costs, the desire for education and culture, and the social frictions arising from urbanisation. Polanyi argued that the 'practical and pragmatic' advance of social legislation responded to the 'objective' needs of industrial societies to manage the 'weaknesses ... inherent in a self-regulating market', a functionalist 'countermove' against 'degradation'.[13] Peacock and Wiseman's long-run study of British public expenditure observed this rising at a far greater rate than GDP, indicating a 'natural ... propensity' of democratic citizens to consume desirable services, compounded by the 'displacement effects' of war, which legitimised state action.[14] New right readings interpreted the same processes first as vote-seeking by cavalier politicians, and later as the errors of socialism, which overturned the successes of capitalist welfare.[15]

The following discussion asks how well this welfare economics model of sectors explains historical transformation in the hospital. Its appropriateness need not be presumed *prima facie*, for its different components were designed to illuminate the present, not to explain change. Despite the accoutrements of social science, such theory was usually developed from assumptions about behaviour rather than empirical testing. Where causation was identified, it was generally in very unspecific terms, evoking broad shifts of majority opinion in liberal democracies. Nonetheless, in what follows it provides a useful heuristic to begin thinking about the problems of growth, change and decline within the three hospital sectors.

Before 1948: patterns of growth and sectoral distribution

The first point to make is that markets do not appear to have prevailed in early hospital provision. In the modern period, the private hospital was most obviously discernible in the area of psychiatric care. By about 1800 surveys of the institutional distribution of 'lunatic' patients showed approximately 200 in private 'madhouses', with some 600 in charitable asylums (the York 'Retreat' for Quakers is the best known), and uncertain numbers in the parish or union workhouses and gaols.[16] It seems plausible that small-scale market operators met demand from families unable to manage insane kin, although many inmates were in fact admitted under contract from Poor Law authorities.[17] The main trend through the nineteenth and early twentieth centuries was the massive expansion of the public sector, following legislation in 1808 to establish rate-funded county asylums. Thenceforth there was a very large rise in the numbers of 'lunatic' admissions—from 477 in 1819-20, to 7,144 in 1850, to 74,004 in 1900—though part of this represented transfers from existing Poor Law accommodation.[18] Private patients were subsequently only a small proportion of the whole: nineteen per cent in 1844, to eleven per cent in 1870 and nine per cent in 1890.[19]

The other manifestation of the public hospital was the infirmary function of the Poor Law workhouse. Parish Poor Law accommodation dates back to the Elizabethan origins of statutorily enshrined localist poor relief. The power to incorporate several parishes to provide a large institution from a broader resource base was originally limited to act of Parliament and thus confined to London and major cities—about fifteen had done so by 1712.[20] Sporadic surveys suggest 129 workhouses were open by 1725, 700 by 1732 and by the 1770s there were some 2,000 institutions, with about 90,000 places.[21] Gilbert's Act of 1782 permitted autonomous combinations of parishes into unions, encouraging more construction. Workhouses accommodated a mix of inmates including the insane, sufferers of infectious diseases, infirm older people, orphaned children, homeless or tramping workers, stigmatised single mothers and the destitute. The mid-nineteenth century saw systematisation through the Poor Law Amendment Act (1834), which created larger administrative 'Unions' and a network of institutions financed by local taxes. The pattern of the mid-century was initially for approvals of general workhouse building with standardised designs, and subsequently for more specialised units, particularly sick wards, within building complexes.[22] Thus, by the early 1900s some workhouses in larger cities had developed as public infirmaries, while others had separate infirmary blocks.

Meanwhile, from the 1870s a network of infectious diseases hospitals emerged, also funded through local property taxes and managed by borough and district councils.[23] These provided isolation facilities for those with notifiable infectious diseases, such as smallpox, scarlet fever, typhoid and diphtheria. In 1929 a Local Government Act carried forward the development of public general hospitals by 'breaking-up' the Poor Law and transferring its functions to local councils, who could then remove the infirmaries from the stigmas of poor relief and manage them as municipal institutions, from which citizens would not be deterred. By 1938, as Table 5.1 shows for England, the public infirmaries—general, poor law or isolation—remained the most important provider in respect of medical care, and also dominated the psychiatric field.

Table 5.1: Numbers and Percentage Distribution of Hospital Beds by Type (excluding asylums) 1861-1938

	1861	1891	1911	1921	1938
Voluntary	14,772	29,520	43,221	56,550	87,235
Public	50,000	83,230	154,273	172,006	175,868
Private		9,500	13,000	26,166	22,547
	%	%	%	%	%
Voluntary	18.51	26.2	21.89	24.75	33.14
Poor Law	81.47	64.71	61.31	52.64	19.94
Local Government		9.16	16.76	22.63	46.89

Source: Robert Pinker, English Hospital Statistics, 61-2; B.Abel-Smith, The Hospitals, 1800-1948, 189

As for the voluntary hospitals, an early wave of foundations in the capitals and provincial cities occurred in the eighteenth century, bringing about sixty general and special hospitals into existence.[24] The endowed trust was superseded as main philanthropic vehicle by this new style subscriber charity, in which donors were issued with admission tickets that they could dispense to applicants (with emergency patients admitted automatically).[25] After 1800 general hospitals opened in most large towns, while specialist institutions (maternity, ophthalmic, ear, nose and throat etc.) followed. Finally, in the late nineteenth and early twentieth century a cottage hospital movement promoted smaller rural institutions.[26] Medical education was supplied at the largest voluntary hospitals, first by honorary consultants providing clinical teaching for apprentices and subsequently through formal links with medical schools.[27] By the early twentieth century, the transition of voluntary hospitals from primarily philanthropic to primarily medical institutions was complete, with the teaching hospitals now major centres of research, laboratory-based diagnosis, clinical training and care.[28]

What about private care? Pay-beds or wards for general medicine were also located in voluntary hospitals, in small numbers, and by the 1930s some had built private blocks as money-making concerns. In London, where these were most numerous, there were 552 paying beds for middle-class patients in 1921, rising to 2,260 by 1938, nearly 11% of the total.[29] This reflected the presence of technical services like radiotherapy and orthopaedic surgery, which removed the social stigma of entering a hospital. By the 1920s there were also considerable numbers of small nursing and maternity homes, with about 26,000 beds.[30] Some were managed by qualified nurses, where eminent doctors attended wealthy patients. Others, prior to licensing legislation (1927), were run by unqualified people, and included centres of complementary healing, rest cures, and 'massage houses'.[31] There was also a trend towards means-tested user fees in the interwar voluntaries, to compensate for the diminution of philanthropic largesse that followed rising tax burdens. However, this was quickly offset by the expansion of mass contributory schemes based principally on small payroll deductions. Given the small scale of the for-profit sector, a private medical insurance system was slow to develop.[32]

How does this first phase fit the specifications of welfare economics for state and voluntarism as reaction for market failure? There seems no evidence that the modern hospital sprang from an inadequate private sector. Nor had that been true of the early or pre-modern hospital. As Guenther Risse's *longue durée* global survey suggests, the hospital has since early times been a 'house of ritual', with its disciplines, daily routines, uniformed staff and ward organisation.[33] Over the very long run, an interplay between religion and the state seems to have been the driver, whether in the sacred settings of Ancient Greek Asclepeiae, or Roman legionary hospitals, or monastic infirmaries, or medieval leper houses, or in the 'hospitals' for orphaned children. An ethic of 'caritas' on the one hand, and on the other the expression of collective purpose by ruling elites, have always mattered most, not the imperative of commerce.

It could however be argued that the new public hospitals responded to a different kind of market failure under early capitalism. Foucault's concept of a 'great confinement' discernible across Europe puts it in simple terms. New spaces of constraint were created by governments—France's *hôpital general*, Britain's workhouse, the German *Zuchthaus*—to house populations defined by their place outside the labour force, including the mad, the sick, the 'beggar', the 'vagabond' and the 'moral libertine'.[34] For Foucault, this was the assertion of 'bourgeois order' through the local arms of the state.[35] The British workhouses, in which public hospital care became embedded, restricted mobility by localising entitlement. Eligibility was also anchored to the complementary 'out-relief' system, providing doles to manage labour market seasonality. More than this though, they represented the liberal creed that poverty amongst working-age adults was moral failing, legitimising crusades against out-relief after 1834 and again in the 1870s.[36] The gradual distinction between the hospital and workhouse function was therefore in part a recognition that sickness caused poverty regardless of character—the germ of the catastrophic costs insight—and so justifiable as both humanity and efficiency.[37] Yet the underlying rationale of separating categories of pauper into deserving and undeserving of aid also meant that as medicalisation proceeded standards tended to be low, with the work disdained by doctors. [38]

The rise of the county asylums also testifies to the default role of the state, rather than the market or charity, in segregating and managing populations unable to negotiate the transition to modernity. Alongside traditional physical restraint, the public asylum adopted new therapeutic routines, which sought to manage insanity in an environment of work, morality and order that instilled social norms and self-control.[39]

Scholarship typically treats the expanding populations of county asylums as a response to rapid urbanisation, which disrupted the solidarities of kinship and community through which emotional distress and psychiatric illness had formerly been dealt.[40] Thus, as fast as the state provided accommodation, so isolated individuals or the families of the insane increased their utilisation—an early manifestation of 'Roemer's Law', that demand for health services tends to follow supply.[41]

What explains the emergence of the British voluntary hospital? In the European context, this was unusual, as elsewhere a single hospital sector that blended philanthropy and public financing was more typical. In part, the voluntary hospital was the obverse of the Poor Law, similarly founded on assessment of entitlement. Its patients were those who merited benevolent support rather than state assistance premised on dependency; here was more forthright acknowledgement that unpredictable and potentially catastrophic illness could impoverish prudent wage-earners. This judgment manifested in the inpatient admission system revolved around obtaining a subscriber's letter from a local dignitary or businessperson. In practice the 'deserving/undeserving' binary was muddy, with quite similar patient populations and voluntary admissions favouring recent in-migrants without a Poor Law settlement or kinship support. Voluntary provision was therefore also a way of managing the labour mobility necessary for economic growth, by prioritising adults of working age with maladies susceptible to cure. [42] The ubiquity of major local employers as donors or subscribers (increasingly through firms rather than as individuals) ought not to be read as kindness alone.[43]

However, it would be reductionist to attribute the voluntary hospital entirely to concerns for human capital and social order. Part of the explanation lies with the supply side: the charitable resources generated by the peculiar combination of factors that underlay British economic dynamism—high agricultural productivity, colonial 'ghost acres' powering trade, finance and services, and the classic industrial revolution in textiles, metals and cheap energy. Also important was the social and political appeal of voluntary association to the urban middle classes.[44] This provided the basis of a new public sphere that undergirded networks of trust, sociability and civic action for both men and women. The personalised admission ticket system also tightened bonds of obligation within hierarchical societies, in ways that the depersonalising Poor Law did not. Finally, because the voluntary hospitals largely accommodated 'deserving' patients with acute diseases, honorary consultants could work in them without loss of social status. Hence it was here that biomedicine became grounded once the Paris revolution in clinical practice diffused outwards, and a more thoroughgoing medicalisation took place.

1942-8 Explaining the critical juncture

For the hospital, the mid-twentieth century establishment of the British NHS marked a distinct break in several respects. The broad parameters of the 1946-7 legislation ensured universal population coverage, comprehensive service provision meeting needs 'from cradle to grave', and progressive tax-funding which rendered access free at the point of use. [45] Within this settlement, voluntary hospitals were 'transferred' from their 'governing body or trustees' and 'vested' in the Minister of Health.[46] Effectively this was compulsion, though hospitals could apply to be 'disclaimed'; 230 were so treated, mostly small religious institutions, hospices and convalescent homes.[47] They now came under the control of appointed statutory bodies, which also oversaw the former Poor Law and local government hospitals. Existing charitable endowments were taken over by the state, although the teaching hospitals retained theirs, with the restriction that they could only be spent on 'non-core NHS' areas: amenities for patients and staff, medical research, and building improvements. Financing came from general taxation, supplemented by a small proportion from national insurance. This built on a growing consensus about the justice of basing state revenue on high levels of income tax, both as a response to the Depression, then to finance the war effort.[48] Along with the demise of locally raised funding went grassroots democracy, hitherto exercised through the local ballot box or on voluntary hospital management committees (which by the 1930s, combined patrician, bourgeois and worker governors).[49] Instead control now resided with the central state, through the accountability of the Minister of Health to Parliament. Private beds were permitted to continue, as a necessary compromise to win professional consent for the reform, but hospital consultants (though not GPs) now became salaried staff.

The short-term narrative of change runs as follows. In the late 1930s a momentum grew amongst health bureaucrats, 'think-tanks', progressive doctors and leftist social reformers in favour of health system reform, with ministerial discussions sparked by funding difficulties in the London teaching hospitals. During wartime, the policy process quickened pace, in response to 'Assumption B' of the Beveridge Report, which stated the necessity of a comprehensive health service within a universalist welfare state. The coalition government introduced proposals for this, including reform of voluntary hospital funding, sidelining charity and mutualism in favour of taxation, and this in turn sharpened debate about how public accountability would follow. The interest groups (doctors, hospital leaders, contributory schemes, local government) disagreed on the optimal arrangements and deadlock ensued. Labour's sweeping victory in 1945 gave Bevan a free hand to override these interests with his bold solution, for in reality only the doctors wielded any political leverage. The BMA was duly pacified with the concession on private beds, and by generous remuneration: GPs remained mostly private contractors to the service, while hospital consultants became salaried. On 5 July 1948, the 'appointed day', the NHS was launched.

Does the welfare economics model, which foregrounds voluntary failure and shifting 'majority opinion', provide an adequate explanation for the hospital settlement? There is good evidence that spatial distribution of voluntary hospital beds was highly uneven, and often inequitable. The 'caprice of charity', in Aneurin Bevan's words, favoured London and wealthy towns like Bath and Oxford, while manifesting an 'inverse care law' of under-resourcing in poor areas like South Wales.[50] However, the pattern of municipal hospital provision was increasingly plugging these gaps, and in this sense a public/voluntary mix still remained viable.[51] Charitable insufficiency also challenged some hospitals. Current account deficits and erosion of capital reserves worsened during the 1930s, as expenditure on staffing, equipment and supplies soared. In part this reflected the inability of middle-class philanthropy to keep pace with patient needs, and although the voluntary sector also generated the solution of mass contributory schemes, these further fueled demand.[52] Again though, financial shortages were limited to particular areas and types of hospital (such as teaching hospitals in London and the North West) and there were also locations where the charity of major donors and community activists remained robust.[53] Bevan also made clear he found voluntary paternalism 'repugnant', and there is some evidence of class resentment at hospital patronage in Mass Observation surveys and diaries.[54] Finally, voluntary particularism was also critiqued in a policy discourse replete with tropes like 'co-ordination', 'integration' and 'co-operation' that highlighted the disjointed nature of the existing provision. Though yoked to greater state agency, this was, paradoxically, a language of the market, derived from industrial management where the vertical integration of the firm similarly promised systematic planning and cost saving.[55]

Beyond this, the case for a shifting social climate in favour of a centralised single-payer system is implicit, not overt. The marked transition of voluntary funding from benevolence to mass contribution (albeit with some charitable overtones) could be read as signalling public acceptance of collective funding, rather than enduring commitment to voluntarism. This was certainly the interpretation of Ministry of Health civil servants.[56] Also heralding change was the demise of the Poor Law, now incorporated within local government, and renamed 'public assistance' to destigmatise access. The idea that consuming public services was a right of citizenship became accepted, and a broad consensus was established around the existing tax and social insurance structure that maintained it.[57] That said though, there is no evidence in contemporary opinion poll data of thirst for reform. On the contrary, most were satisfied with the existing mixed economy, and this only changed somewhat in 1942-5 after the Beveridge Report was disseminated.[58]

In sum, while the welfare economics model provides context for the NHS system change, its evidence is too ambiguous to offer a fundamental explanation. Other causes were contingent, such as the effect of the Second World War, ratcheting the pace of state action through the creation of an Emergency Medical Service. This empowered government to manage the whole hospital sector to cope with civilian and military war casualties, stabilising hospital finances, rationalising labour flows, and accustoming the population to public control.[59] Another relevant consideration is the role of the labour movement. The comparative historiography, pointing for example to the Scandinavian and New Zealand experience, argues that in periods of social democratic party-political control, welfare policy will be more generous and expansive.[60] To the extent that the NHS was the creation of a majority Labour government, and Bevan himself a left-wing tribune schooled in the coalminers' union, this has some salience. But again, it is an incomplete account. Much of the reform process had occurred earlier, under the cross-party wartime coalition government.

Moreover, while some socialists and trade unionists clearly advocated public provision, Britain's labour movement had no unitary position.[61] Many trade unionists were also voluntary hospital worker governors, content with the status quo; others favoured extending coverage through social insurance, not taxation; and the left generally envisaged a local government health service, not one under the central state.[62]

A final aspect of this complex web of causes is the 'institutionalist' analysis, which argues that the nature of the state and the legislative process is the key determinant.[63] The British state had several features that facilitated radical change. It was essentially a two-party system, where elections periodically delivered the winner a strong governing majority, where legislative proposals came predominantly from Cabinet, where members' loyalty to the party whip was the norm, and where law making was unhampered by an obstructive second chamber or a complex committee system. Also in play were path-dependent processes—in the sense of former policy decisions that shaped later trajectories. In particular, the early introduction of national health insurance (NHI) in 1911 had accustomed much of the population to state entitlements, while raising expectations for their expansion (not least to include hospital coverage).[64] NHI had also undermined the opposition of the British Medical Association. Formed in 1832, since the 1890s this had functioned increasingly as the doctor's trade union, initially defending their interests as friendly society employees.[65] Though vocally opposing the NHS proposals, its membership proved more amenable, having experienced the personal economic advantages of state provision since 1911. Probably ministers also concluded that apparently implacable hostility was just sabre-rattling.

A narrow welfare economics explanation therefore furnishes only part of the context for the coming of Britain's NHS, and the consequent impact on hospitals. Other contributing factors were the impact of war, the position of labour and the conducive institutional setting, and last but not least, the electoral mathematics favouring the Atlee government.[66]

1948-2010 The changing pattern of hospital provision and utilisation

In the NHS era, the pattern of sectoral distribution had changed, such that hospitals were now predominantly public institutions. Initially only limited private provision remained under the new dispensation, although, as Table 5.2 illustrates, it was soon to grow.

Table 5.2: Private Medicine under the NHS, UK 1955-2009

	Private Medical Insurance		Independent Acute Hospitals		
	Subscribers	Population			Private spend
	000s	Coverage %	Hospitals	Beds	as % UK total
1955	274	1.2			
1960	467	1.9			
1965	680	2.7			
1970	930	3.6			
1975	1,087	4.1			
1980	1,647	6.4	154	7,035	
1985	2,380	8.9	200	9,955	9.9
1990	3,300	11.7	211	10,739	15.9
1995	3,430	11.4	227	11,681	19.8
2000	3,664	11.7	225	9,980	19
2005	3,511	106	213	9,578	16.4
2009	3,3,425	9.7	213	9,366	15.8

Source: Laing's Healthcare Market Review 2010-2011, 36, 58, 144

It had survived a fierce debate when the Labour government (1974-9) sought to phase out pay beds in NHS hospitals. Not only did this boost separate private hospital foundations, it also failed in its own terms, with NHS pay beds first falling from 4,919 (1974) to 2,819 (1981), then rising to 3,144 by 1983, following legislation reinstituting NHS consultants' rights to private practice.[67] Private hospital expansion of capacity also followed the fostering of commercial medical insurance by government from the 1980s. Insurance companies such as BUPA and Medicash were descendants of the contributory scheme movement, initially retaining a non-profit stance and socially responsible ethics.[68] Another pre-war philanthropic foundation, the Nuffield Trust, became a significant hospital provider outside the NHS. Other private insurers and hospitals were more purely commercial, and their presence in the British medical market was aided in the 1990s and 2000s by the liberalisation of international trade in services, promoted by the European Union and the World Trade Organisation.[69] More recently, a policy of encouraging NHS commissioners to consider 'any qualified provider' when tendering for services opened further opportunities for sectoral growth.

The other main pattern of change, shown in Table 5.3, lay within the public sector. This was the relative decline of the hospital as a locus of health care, in favour of primary and community settings. The downward trend of utilisation, and the accompanying reduction in bed numbers was visible first and most markedly in the psychiatric hospitals. Here volumes began a sequential decline from the 1950s, which continued in the 1960s, after the then Minister of Health, Enoch Powell, inaugurated a closure policy. A famous speech conjured grim imagery of the asylum: 'isolated, majestic, imperious, brooded over by the gigantic water-tower ... rising unmistakable and daunting out of the countryside'.[70] Part of the aim was to incorporate psychiatric units in new general hospitals proposed by the 1962 Hospital Plan,

Table 5.3: NHS hospital beds and inpatients, 1951—2009/10

	All				Mental Health	
	Beds	Beds	Beds	Beds	Inpatients	Beds
	Eng & Wa	UK	Eng & Wa	UK	Eng & Wa	Eng
	'000s	'000s	Per 1,000 population		'000s	'000s
1951	467	543	10.7	10.8	145*	
1955	482	561	10.8	11	151**	
1960	479	560	10.5	10.7	135***	
1965	470	551	9.9	10.1	124	
1970	456	536	9.3	9.6	103	
1975	419	497	8.5	8.8		
1980	383	458	7.7	8.1		
1985	348	422	7	7.5		67
1990/1	274	338	5.4	5.9		55
1995/6	222	273	4.3	4.7		39
2000/01	201	242	3.8	4.1		34
2005/06	189	226	3.5	3.7		30
2010/11	155	186	2.8	3		23

Source: E. Hawe and L. Cockcroft, OHE Guide to UK Health and Health Care Statistics, London: Office of Health Economics, 2013, 102; Kathleen Jones, History of the Mental Health Services, 358-9; Ewbank, Thompson, McKenna, NHS Hospital Bed Numbers, Figure 4. *1949 **1954 ***1961

further medicalising a field that had hitherto blended treatment with control. Partly it was to devolve greater duties of care to local authority welfare departments, increasingly staffed by professional social workers. This policy accelerated in the 1980s when it was framed as a transition to 'care in the community'.[71]

Also underlying the numerical decline of the public hospital were changes to general health care. The post-war development of geriatric medicine as a specialty had reduced hospitalisation of the older infirm. These were patients who had hitherto been abandoned to the 'therapeutic nihilism' of the residential or infirmary wards of Poor Law institutions, where low staffing and skill levels militated against active treatment.[72] Now bed throughput levels rose, and length of stay declined, again benefitting from the extension of community services such as home helps, home nursing and 'meals-on-wheels' (originally a wartime innovation). Over time the material fabric of the Poor Law legacy was replaced by new hospitals and old peoples' homes (though many sturdy ex-workhouses and asylums enjoy postmodern afterlife as residential housing or business centres).[73] Technological and surgical changes also reduced the length of time spent in acute hospital beds. Numerical decline has been long-term, since a peak in the early 1960s. Between 1979 and 2012 there has been there been an overall decline of 59%. This was composed of a 35% fall in acute beds, with much larger reductions in geriatric (65%), psychiatric (74%), and maternity (58%) beds, hardly offset by a small rise in numbers of day beds (for very short stays) to 8.7% of the total bed stock by 2016/17.[74]

What can the welfare economics model contribute to explaining these different patterns? A 'state failure' argument was certainly introduced by proponents of private hospitals, initially in response to empirical evidence of two areas of difficulty for the NHS—waiting lists, which were held to be caused by the moral hazard inherent in a free service, which produced excess demand, and the continuing spatial inequities of funding, beds and specialist care, which the reform still had not alleviated by the 1960s.[75] In the 1980s, as enthusiasm rose for privatisation, it was suggested these shortcomings might be obviated by commercialising hospital care, so that the price mechanism would adjust supply to demand more effectively.[76] Conversely, as Thatcherite austerity restrained public expenditure, the argument changed. Now it was proposed that fostering private hospitals would ease the burden of state insufficiency, by siphoning well-heeled patients off towards comfortable paying hospitals; this justified generous tax treatment for private insurance.[77] Subsequently, as NHS commissioning from the private sector increased, initially for ancillary services, and more recently for medical care, the emphasis changed again. Now the focus was on the greater efficiencies that a private hospital should be able to achieve, thanks to the spur of the profit motive so lacking in state institutions.[78]

The empirical evidence underpinning all this has been ambiguous and hampered by poor data. In the 2000s, economists evaluated the results of NHS contracting from 'independent sector treatment centres' (ISTCs). Critics had worried about 'cream-skimming', whereby ISTCs concentrated on less challenging procedures from which it was easier to make profit, thus leaving the NHS with more difficult, costly cases. There was some evidence for this, alongside the perceived benefits of driving down waiting lists.[79] More recently there have been claims that health outcomes were better in regions where commissioners have the greatest choice of alternative public and private providers; it is hypothesised that this is because competition has galvanised hospital managers to greater efforts. However, the outcome data are limited, the underlying regressions based on imperfect mapping of hospital catchments onto mortality data, and the causal pathways uncertain.[80] In sum, the survival and growth of the private sector needs to be understood less in terms of its positive attributes *vis a vis* state failure. More important has been the political context in which it has operated, with accommodation from the left and positive encouragement from the right.

What about the numerical decline of hospital beds? Neither state failure, nor state successes seem particularly apposite as explanations. Dehospitalisation has been a feature of all advanced industrial economies, with the reasons primarily located in technological change, the greater efficiency of surgical procedures and pharmaceutical therapies, particularly of psychiatric illness. It is certainly arguable that British deinstitutionalisation has gone comparatively further and faster: in 2004, for example, the UK had about 3 acute beds per 1,000 population, whereas European peers like Belgium (7 per 1,000), Germany (6.5) and France (4.7) had more. Given that these nations had mixed insurance modes of health funding and plural hospital ownership, then it may be that the tendency of the single-payer NHS towards greater cost-containment has been a factor.[81] However, whether or not this has made the system relatively more vulnerable to shortages is dependent on other factors, such as the availability of social care accommodation, and the quality of treatment in primary and community settings.

With respect to psychiatric beds, the asylum's demise has been much debated by historians of madness. Their main focus has been on the medications that have underlain deinstitutionalisation, beginning with the antipsychotic chlorpromazine in the 1950s, and subsequently antidepressants.[82] Some countered this technological account with an emphasis on political economy. Was the real motive for Powell's 'water tower' speech a desire for a cheaper model of managing the disorderly nature of mental illness? Similar suspicions fuelled the critique of late twentieth-century community care. A cognate argument is that rather than providing a chemical 'cure', drug therapies work by altering intellectual and emotional processes in potentially harmful ways.[83] At its demise, the asylum has also had its champions, who elegised its humanitarian achievement in providing refuge and care. However, it would be difficult to conclude from all this that the imperative of restraining expenditure was distinctive to the statist NHS.[84] 'Decarceration' and the accompanying anti-psychiatry movement was a widespread phenomenon, spanning for example Basaglia in Italy, Foucault in France, Szasz, Goffmann, Kesey in the USA, and Laing in Scotland. If its common theme was state failure, then this was within a larger argument about the harmful effects of social control.

Finally, sociology provides another account of the hospitals' demise that is rooted in the concept of medicalisation and neutral towards sectoral type.[85] This begins from the argument that the hospital's long run transformation from refuge to clinic was a timebound phenomenon. As medicine staked a claim to knowledge based on pathology and bacteriology, spaces were needed in which medical practitioners had bodies readily available for analysis. By the mid-twentieth century, the status of biomedicine was assured, and with the decline of infectious disease the clinical gaze began to turn outside the hospital's walls and into the community.[86] The cancers and cardio-vascular diseases appeared to have preclinical causes, rooted in individual choices about behaviour and consumption, long preceding their morbid manifestation. The result was an increasing medicalisation of society itself, in which a 'surveillance medicine' sought to turn unhealthy consumers into virtuous self-governing subjects.[87] Whether this claim has any predictive power remains to be seen. The secular decline of hospital capacity has certainly continued since it was enunciated, although the rate has slowed markedly since 2010. The advantages for fixed costs of concentrating expertise in large institutions seem likely to persist. For example, the long run retreat from home births in favour of increasingly large hospital obstetric units remains almost complete, despite the safety advantage now having disappeared (proportion of births at home: 1927—85%; 1948—46%; 1965—28%; 1981—1%; 2010–2.5%).[88]

1948 to 2010: NHS hospitals under the state—success or failure?

In arguing for the NHS, Bevan had claimed that centralising and nationalising the hospital system would eradicate the inequities of access determined by place and local prosperity. It would universalise the best, bring serenity 'in place of fear' and deliver efficient, effective care.[89] The assumption behind this, and in the policy documents that had informed the debate, was that system integration under responsible administrative bodies, coupled with stable financing, would inevitably bring this about. How well did the public hospitals perform in the era of control by the central state?

Before attempting a general appraisal, it is important to note that hospital policy-making, however good or bad, took place within a budgetary envelope set from above. With charity now consigned to marginal areas, and income from the pay beds minimal, the scope of activity was determined by the annual financial settlement. In almost every year since 1948, this Exchequer subvention for the NHS included a real increase. However, as is well known, the rising proportion of older people in the population, and hence the overall prevalence of morbidity, has driven a commensurate rise in demand. Technological costs and culturally determined expectations of service have also fuelled this. However, the pace of real increase to the NHS budget has been quite variable over time, with three periods—the early 1950s, the 1980s-1990s, and the 2010s—times of relative austerity.[90] All three periods have been episodes of Conservative government, in which NHS expenditure played second fiddle to broader economic policy considerations.

International comparison also casts light on the financial constraints within which hospital policy must be judged. As in Table 5.4, this consistently shows British health expenditure to have been relatively modest when set against peer nations, whether viewed in real per capita terms, or as a proportion of GDP.

Table 5.4: Current health expenditure (public and private) as share (%) of gross domestic product, UK and comparator nations

	1970	1980	1990	2000	2010	2017
France	5.2	6.7	8.0	9.5	11.2	11.5
Germany	5.7	8.1	8.0	9.8	11.0	11.3
Japan	4.4	6.2	5.8	7.2	9.2	10.7
Sweden	5.5	7.8	7.3	7.4	8.5	10.9
United Kingdom	4.0	5.1	5.1	6.0	8.5	9.6
United States	6.2	8.2	11.3	12.5	16.4	17.2

Source: OECD. Stat URL: https://stats.oecd.org/Index.aspx?DataSetCode=SHA# 19 May 2019

Two conclusions are possible. One is that the NHS model has been particularly suitable for maximising efficiency and preventing waste. The other is that this kind of single payer, centralised system has been more vulnerable to under-funding than those based on social insurance (Germany, Japan), local taxation (Sweden), or plural sources (United States). Until the 1990s, comparative health outcome data was limited and tended to support the former; since then however, Britain's poor ranking against indicators like avoidable mortality and cancer survival rates has inclined judgment to the latter.[91] If so, then it is here that the real 'state failure' of the NHS model lies, with its 'institutionalised parsimony' and vulnerability to Conservative retrenchment. [92]

The financial constraints of the 1950s explain the initial difficulties faced by the NHS hospitals, when regional health boards (RHBs) and their subsidiary hospital management boards (HMBs) found themselves unable to implement development plans due to lack of resources. Indeed, capital expenditure in the 1950s ran at a lower level than in the 1930s. This though is explicable in terms of post-war austerity, when social spending on health took second place to that on council housing and school building. Within this context the newly integrated management structure did nonetheless deliver some achievements. Annual accounting became standardised and systematic. Savings from fixed costs for energy and laundries, and from bulk order of food and supplies, could now be obtained by HMBs, which mostly contained a cluster of hospitals. Regional treasurers monitored comparative costings and alerted institutions to areas of potential waste. Clinical management committees planned the distribution of specialists within the region, ensuring that expertise became better allocated in light of estimated need (though inter-regional disparities remained).[93] Alongside this came the capacity to manage the overall hospital stock, for example to further the goals of geriatric medicine, or to repurpose the increasingly redundant infectious diseases hospitals.

State direction became more ambitious in the 1960s under Enoch Powell's Hospital Plan. In addition to the asylum closures, planning sought to establish optimum bed to patient ratios, then to meet these through a network of district general hospitals, which would combine acute, geriatric, psychiatric and other specialty beds. Historical verdicts have been unkind to the Plan, though for its execution rather than its ambition. It transpired that Britain had neither the building capacity, nor sufficient technical expertise, nor the sustained public investment capital to support the programme, and much went unfulfilled.[94] A further problem followed the reduction of geriatric beds (based on a contestable ratio), which was made without proper reference to the capacity of social care in local government to provide complementary services. This was where the 'bed-blocking' phenomenon began, as the NHS vied with local authorities to shunt infirm patients, and their associated costs, across the imprecise health/social care boundary.[95] Here the problem was not state failure per se, but rather Bevan's decision to create bespoke administrative structures for the NHS, instead of situating hospitals within local government, where they would have sat alongside community care.

Faith in statist system planning continued into the 1970s, when the problem of spatial inequity was finally tackled by the 'RAWP'—a population-based formula for allocating funding to the regions and subsidiary districts. This was politically controversial for it meant moving resources away from the traditionally well-funded regions of London and the Home Counties to the provinces. The mid-1970s also saw a more concerted attempt to improve equity between different areas of the NHS, for the 'Cinderella services' of geriatrics and mental health had hitherto received disproportionately less funding than acute medicine. The programme budgeting initiative began an incremental adjustment towards those areas, again in response to a calculus of need. In both cases this represented successful, decisive action to overturn a stasis built into the system by history, and it did not emerge *deus ex machina* from state processes. It depended on conviction leadership by Labour politicians Barbara Castle and David Owen, and also on the emergence of experts able to frame and implement highly technical policy.[96]

From the 1980s a raft of policies was introduced that explicitly invoked state failure in their justification. The early Thatcher governments sought to improve efficiency and cost effectiveness by introducing management techniques from the private sector, and by treating patients more as customers whose wishes and needs merited more attention. Notions of 'provider capture' were expressed by theoreticians of the new public management, though the political discourse was more focused on resolving unstable industrial relations and upping productivity. First came the principles of Rayner scrutinies—target setting, and holding regional heads to account—coupled with the Korner health informatics initiatives. Next was the Griffiths

Report, inaugurating the replacement of consensual decision-making by general management under a single leader. A related attempt to import a new cadre of managers from the business world was only partially successful.[97]

Then in 1991 came the 'internal market', and a more decisive step away from a vertically managed, statist hospital system. The idea was to create a hybrid structure, which retained state ownership and financing, but mimicked market dynamics. It did so by obliging hospitals to price and sell their services to purchasing bodies, at first mainly in the form of regional and local health authorities, but increasingly of locally clustered primary care providers. The New Labour government retained this model, though replaced the language of 'purchasing' with 'commissioning'. This acknowledged the reality that there was little actual 'market' competition, because in most places purchasing was monopsonistic, and providing monopolistic. Gradually this was modified through ISTCs and what came to be called the 'any qualified provider' scheme, which encouraged commissioning from private sector bodies. Commerce was also to be the engine of capital improvement, with a 'private finance initiative' (PFI) now the norm for new building. This operated through government agreeing long-term contracts with private companies to build and manage hospitals, and resulted in a rapid expansion and renovation of the stock in the Blair/Brown years.

Has the performance of NHS hospitals under this policy regime borne out the driving assumptions of state failure and market strengths? The evidence is mixed. The new public management reforms of the 1980s did not prevent a growing public sense of crisis (arguably driven by underfunding) that in turn propelled the late Thatcher government towards more radical change.[98] Nor did early evaluations of the internal market show strong evidence of greater productivity. Part of the problem was that commissioning was complex and difficult, with the advantages of price information lying on the providers' side; also, its total cost within the system was opaque, rendering a historical cost/benefit appraisal impossible.[99] Considerable criticism has also been directed against PFI, which locked taxpayers into some costly and disadvantageous contracts, just as innovative approaches were moving care out of hospitals. As for patient satisfaction, public opinion data shows that this has moved closely in step with funding levels, not structural reform, rising significantly during the Blair years as Labour increased inputs.[100] All that said though, commissioning has become settled policy, and medical professionals generally approve the empowerment of primary care on the one hand, and the greater cost-consciousness of hospitals on the other.

It should also be noted that alongside this incorporation of market dynamics has been a strengthening of the state's armoury of control over doctors. The National Institute of Clinical Excellence (NICE) was established in 1997 to approve drugs and therapies, constraining liberty of prescription and treatment.[101] This was accompanied by Clinical Framework Guidelines, which sought to standardise activities according to best practice. The use of targets and published league tables of hospital activity was the state's effort to incentivise improvement through 'naming and shaming'; the initial use of this strategy in England seemed to be delivering results, but later research suggested no sustained effect.[102] Similarly, hospitals now had to accept the publication of 'patient reported outcome measures', which revealed success rates of different procedures. Finally, although the 2012 Health and Social Care Act attempted to remove the last vestiges of hierarchical administration, this quickly proved unsuccessful. The aim was to abolish regional authorities, so that the hospital trusts and 'clinical commissioning groups' would become free agents, operating mostly autonomously, with only light touch regulation from the central state.[103] Yet almost immediately regional authorities had to be reinvented as Structural Transformation Plan areas.[104] Integrated planning, it transpired, was necessary after all.

In sum, although state failure was much invoked in recent years, the evidence for its existence is not compelling. Moreover, administrative and political preference led the British to retain a statist system, but seek to improve it by making it more responsive to price and demand. Again, it is not very clear whether these strategies have really achieved their goal. In 2010, as New Labour faltered, NHS indicators of productivity, waiting times and satisfaction were all extremely positive.[105] However, it remains perfectly plausible that this is explained by the sustained funding increases of 2000-2010, rather than by the internal market model of the Blair/Brown years.

Conclusion

The main focus of this discussion has been the changing balance of the public, private and voluntary sectors in the history of the British hospital. It has interrogated a conceptual model drawn from the welfare economics literature which proposed that each sector has certain attributes. The hypothesis was that in the medical field, there are some things that the private hospital can do well, but other things it does badly, and so too for the voluntary and the public hospital. To explain change then, we might confirm empirically the existence of these attributes, then look for evidence of shifts in opinion about their relative desirability.

In applying this model to the long-run pattern of change it does seem to offer some helpful insight, at least based on the British case. For example, there was the historic marginality of the private hospital, initially important in mental health care, but quickly superseded, and retaining only a small share of general hospital activity, including under the NHS, when it served wealthier individuals seeking greater comfort or speedier attention. Instead, the state and voluntary sectors were always dominant in hospital provision, because some form of collective arrangement was needed to regulate financing, above and beyond an individual's capacity to pay fees. The state's importance was in marshalling resources for marginal groups that sickness had cast outside the labour market, and whose distress needed to be managed, for reasons of humanity and social stability. The voluntary hospital emerged to provide care for sick people within the labour market, and was less discriminatory.

However, the welfare economics framework did not seem sufficient to explain moments of significant political transition, other than as general context. Instead, to reach a satisfactory account of change was to acknowledge more complex patterns of causation, in which social and political history mattered as well as economic. This raises the question of whether the positivist claims on which the model draws are valid. Instead perhaps its assumptions about inherent attributes are chimera—either descriptions of transitory phenomena, or normative judgments? International comparison should provide further insight into this question, and hence into whether this way of conceptualising the hospital sectors is useful for understanding historical change.

1. John V. Pickstone, Medicine and Industrial Society: A History of Hospital Development in Manchester and Its Region : 1752-1946 (Manchester: Manchester University Press, 1985); Brian Abel-Smith, The Hospitals, 1800-1948; a Study in Social Administration in England and Wales (London: Heinemann, 1964).

2. Adam Smith, An Inquiry into the Nature and Causes of the Wealth of Nations (Chicago: University of Chicago Press, 1977 [1776]), 593.

3. Daniel Tarschys, 'The Growth of Public Expenditures: Nine Modes of Explanation', Scandinavian Political Studies, 10, A10 (1975), 9–31; Adolph Wagner, Grundlegung der politischen Oekonomie, (3rd. edn.1893 [1876]), reproduced in, C.J. Bullock, Selected Readings in Public Finance (Boston: Ginn and co, 1906, 2nd edn 1920), 32.

4. Alan Williams, 'Primeval Health Economics in Britain: Personal Retrospect on the Pre-HESG Period', Health Economics, 7 (1998), S3–8; K. Arrow, 'Uncertainty and the Welfare Economics of Medical Care', American Economic Review, 53, 5 (1963), 941-973; Nicholas Barr, The Economics of the Welfare State (Oxford: Oxford University Press, 1998), 78-88.

5. G. Finlayson, Citizen, State and Social Welfare in Britain (Oxford: Oxford University Press, 1994), 287-8.

6. Elizabeth Macadam, The New Philanthropy: A Study in the Relations Between the Statutory and Voluntary Social Services (London: Allen & Unwin, 1934), 33, 49, 113, 296-9; C. Braithwaite, The Voluntary Citizen, an Enquiry into the Place of Philanthropy in the Community (London: Methuen, 1938); A.F.C. Bourdillon (ed), Voluntary Social Services: Their Place in the Modern State (London: Methuen, 1945).

7. F.S. Nitti, 'General Survey and Interpretation of the Facts', in Bullock, op. cit. (note 3), 46.

8. B. Weisbrod, 'Towards a theory of the Voluntary Nonprofit Sector in a Three Sector Economy', in E. S. Phelps (ed), Altruism, Morality and Economic Theory (New York: Russell Sage Foundation, 1975); L. Salamon, Partners in Public Service: Government-Nonprofit Relations in the Modern Welfare State (London: Johns Hopkins, 1995).

9. William Niskanen, Bureaucracy and Representative Government (Chicago: Adline, 1971).

10. Gordon Tullock, 'The Welfare Costs of Tariffs, Monopolies, and Theft', Western Economic Journal, 5, 3 (1967), 224-32; Anne O. Krueger, 'The Political Economy of the Rent-Seeking Society', American Economic Review, 64, 3 (1974), 291-303.

11. Julian Le Grand, Motivation, Agency, and Public Policy: Of Knights and Knaves, Pawns and Queens (Oxford: Oxford University Press, 2006), 57.

12. Albert O. Hirschman, Exit, Voice, and Loyalty: Responses to Decline in Firms, Organizations, and States (Cambridge, MA: Harvard University Press,1970).

13. Karl Polanyi, The Great Transformation:

the political and economic origins of our time (Boston, Beacon Press, 1944, 2nd edn, 2001), 41, 152-4, 160.

14. A. Peacock and J. Wiseman The Growth of Public Expenditure in the United Kingdom (London: Allen & Unwin, 2nd, edn 1967 [1961]).

15. Arthur Seldon, The Virtues of Capitalism (Indianapolis: Liberty Fund, 2004), 310-41.

16. Chris Philo, A Geographical History of Institutional Provision for the Insane from Medieval Times to the 1860s in England and Wales. The Space Reserved for Insanity (Lampeter: Edwin Mellen Press, 2004); the binary 'able-bodied/non-able-bodied in contemporary surveys was extremely imprecise, see J.D. Marshall, The Old Poor Law, 1795-1834 (London: Macmillan, 1968).

17. Peter Bartlett, The Poor Law of Lunacy: The Administration of Pauper Lunatics in Mid-Nineteenth-Century England (London: Leicester University Press, 1999), 37.

18. Philo, op. cit. (note 16), 354; Kathleen Jones, A History of the Mental Health Services, London: Routledge and Kegan Paul, 1972, 357.

19. Andrew Scull, Museums of Madness: The Social Organization of Insanity in Nineteenth-Century England, London: Allen Lane, 1979, 244.

20. Lynn Hollen Lees, The Solidarities of Strangers: The English Poor Laws and the People, 1700-1948 (Cambridge: Cambridge University Press, 1998), 61.

21. Paul Slack, The English Poor Law, 1531-1782 (Cambridge: Cambridge University Press, ed. 1995), 34; Lees, op. cit. (note 20), 61.

22. Felix Driver, Power and Pauperism: The Workhouse System, 1834-1844 (Cambridge: Cambridge University Press, 1993), 78.

23. M.L. Newsom Kerr, Contagion, Isolation, and Biopolitics in Victorian London (Cham: Palgrave Macmillan, 2017).

24. M. Gorsky, J. Mohan, M. Powell, 'British Voluntary Hospitals, 1871–1938: The Geography of Provision and Utilization', Journal of Historical Geography, 25, 4 (1999), 463–482, 466.

25. R. Porter, 'The Gift Relation: Philanthropy and Provincial Hospitals in Eighteenth Century England', in L. Granshaw and R. Porter, eds., The Hospital in History (London, 1989) 149-78; Abel-Smith, op. cit. (note 1), 4-15.

26. S. Cherry, 'Change and Continuity in the Cottage Hospitals c. 1859-1948', Medical History, 36 (1992) 271-89

27. Abel-Smith, op. cit. (note 1).

28. K. Waddington, Charity and the London Hospitals, 1850-1898 (Woodbridge: Boydell and Brewer, 2000); S. Sturdy and R. Cooter, 'Science, scientific management and the transformation of medicine in Britain, 1870-1950', History of Science, xxxvi (1998), 421-66.

29. King Edward's Hospital Fund for London, Statistical Summary ... for the Year 1921, London: King Edward's Hospital

Fund for London, 1922, 16-20, King Edward's Hospital Fund for London, Statistical Summary ... for the Year 1938, London: King Edward's Hospital Fund for London, 1939, 86; there were 20,973 beds in the London voluntaries in 1938, see Pinker, English Hospitals, 81.

30. Abel-Smith, op. cit. (note 1), 339.

31. Abel-Smith, op. cit. (note 1), 191, 339-45.

32. M. Gorsky & J. Mohan with T. Willis Mutualism and health care: British hospital contributory schemes in the twentieth-century (Manchester, Manchester University Press, 2006).

33. Guenter Risse, Mending bodies, saving souls: a history of hospitals (Oxford: Oxford University Press, 1999), 5-9.

34. Michel Foucault, Madness and Civilization: a history of insanity in the age of reason (London: Routledge, 1993 [1967]), 38-64.

35. Foucault, op. cit. (note 34), 55, 58.

36. Karel Williams, From Pauperism to Poverty (London: Routledge & Kegan Paul, 1981).

37. Anne Digby, Pauper Palaces (London: Routledge & Kegan Paul, 1978).

38. M.A. Crowther, The Workhouse System, the History of an English Social Institution (London: Methuen, 1981), 156–75; Martin Gorsky, 'Creating the Poor Law Legacy: Institutional Care for Older People Before the Welfare State', Contemporary British History, 26, 4 (2012), 441-465.

39. Foucault, op. cit. (note 34), 241-76.

40. John Walton, 'Lunacy in the Industrial Revolution': A Study of Asylum Admissions in Lancashire, 1848-50', Journal of Social History, 13, 1 (1979), 1-22; Andrew Scull, Museums of Madness: The Social Organization of Insanity in Nineteenth-Century England (Harmondsworth: Penguin, 1982).

41. M. Shain, M.I. Roemer, 'Hospital costs relate to the supply of beds', Modern Hospital, 92, 4 (1959), 71–3.

42. M.E. Fissell, Patients, Power and Poor in Eighteenth Century Bristol (Cambridge: Cambridge University Press, 1991); J. Woodward, To Do the Sick No Harm (London: Routledge and Kegan Paul, 1974), 36-74

43. M. Gorsky, Patterns of Philanthropy, Charity and Society in Nineteenth-Century Bristol (Woodbridge: Boydell and Brewer, 1999); F. Prochaska, The Voluntary Impulse: Philanthropy in Modern Britain (London: Faber & Faber, 1988), xiii-xiv.

44. R. Porter 'The gift relation: philanthropy and provincial hospitals in eighteenth-century England', in L. Granshaw and R. Porter (eds) The Hospital in History (London: Routledge, 1989), 149-78; A. Wilson 'Conflict, Consensus and Charity: Politics and the Provincial Voluntary Hospitals in the Eighteenth Century' English Historical Review cxi, 442 (1996), 599-619; A. Borsay '"Persons of Honour and Reputation" The Voluntary Hospital in an Age of Corruption' Medical History, 35,(1991), 281-294; M. Gorsky, Patterns of Philanthropy, Charity and Society in Nineteenth-Century Bristol (Woodbridge: Boydell and Brewer, 1999); R.J. Morris, Class,

Sect and Party: The Making of the British Middle Class: Leeds, 1820-50 (Manchester: Manchester University Press, 1990).

45. C. Webster, The Health Services since the War, Vol. 1, Problems of Health Care: The National Health Service before 1957 (London: HMSO, 1988); C. Webster,The National Health Service: A Political History (Oxford: Oxford University Press, 2002 [1998]); R. Klein, The New Politics of the NHS: From Creation to Reinvention (Oxford: Radcliffe Publishing, 2006 [1983]).

46. National Health Service Act, 1946. 9 & 10 Geo. 6 Ch. 81, Section 6, 4

47. Joan Higgins, The Business of Medicine: Private Health Care in Britain (Basingstoke: Macmillan Education, 1988), 19, 22.

48. Martin Daunton, Just Taxes: The Politics of Taxation in Britain (Cambridge: Cambridge University Press, 2007).

49. Martin Gorsky, 'Community involvement in hospital governance in Britain: evidence from before the National Health Service', International Journal of Health Services, 4 (2008), 751-771; Gorsky, Mohan, Willis, op. cit. (note 32).

50. M. Gorsky, J. Mohan, and M. Powell, 'British Voluntary Hospitals, 1871–1938: The Geography of Provision and Utilization', Journal of Historical Geography, 25 (1999), 463–82; Julian Tudor Hart, 'The Inverse Care Law', The Lancet, 297, 7696 (1971), 405-412.

51. John Mohan, 'The Caprice of Charity: Regional Variations in Finances of British Voluntary Hospitals, c. 1891–1944', in

M. Gorsky and S. Sheard(eds) Financing Medicine: The British Experience (London: Routledge, 2006), 77–92.

52. M. Gorsky, J. Mohan & M. Powell, 'The Financial Health of Voluntary Hospitals in Interwar Britain', Economic History Review, 55, 3 (2002), 533–57.

53.N. Hayes & B.M. Doyle, 'Eggs, Rags and Whist Drives: Popular Munificence and the Development of Provincial Medical Voluntarism Between the Wars', Historical Research, 86, 234 (2013), 712–740; N. Hayes, 'Our Hospitals'? Voluntary Provision, Community and Civic Consciousness in Nottingham Before the NHS', Midland History, 37, 1 (2012), 84–105.

54. Higgins, op. cit. (note 47), 27; Mass Observation Archive, 'Attitudes to State Medicine', 1943; Diarist 5378, 992; N. Hayes, 'Did We Really Want a National Health Service? Hospitals, Patients and Public Opinions before 1948', English Historical Review, cxxvii, 526 (2012), 625-61.

55. L. Hannah, The Rise of the Corporate Economy (London: Methuen, 1976), 123-30, 139-40; Sturdy and Cooter, 'Science, scientific management', 425-30.

56. M. Gorsky, J. Mohan & T. Willis, 'Hospital contributory schemes and the NHS debates 1937-46: the rejection of social insurance in the British welfare state?' Twentieth Century British History, 16, 2 (2005), 170-92.

57. M.J. Daunton, 'Payment and Participation: Welfare and State-Formation in Britain 1900–1951', Past & Present, 150, 1 (1996), 169–216.

58. Hayes, op. cit. (note 54).

59. Richard M. Titmuss, Problems of Social Policy (London: H.M.S.O, 1950).

60. Francis G. Castles, The Social Democratic Image of Society: A Study of the Achievements and Origins of Scandinavian Social Democracy in Comparative Perspective (London: Routledge & Kegan Paul, 1978); Gøsta Esping-Andersen, The Three Worlds of Welfare Capitalism (Cambridge: Polity Press, 2012).

61. B.M. Doyle, 'Labour and Hospitals in Urban Yorkshire: Middlesbrough, Leeds and Sheffield, 1919–1938', Social History of Medicine 23 (2010), 374–392; Barry Doyle, The Politics of Hospital Provision in Early Twentieth-Century Britain (London: Pickering and Chatto, 2014).

62. John Stewart, The Battle for Health: A Political History of the Socialist Medical Association, 1930-51 (Aldershot: Ashgate, 1999).

63. E. Immergut, Health Politics: Interests and Institutions in Western Europe (Cambridge: Cambridge University Press, 1992).

64. J.S. Hacker, 'The Historical Logic of National Health Insurance: Structure and Sequence in the Development of British, Canadian, and U.S. Medical Policy', Studies in American Political Development, 12 (1998), 57–130.

65. Andrew Morrice, 'Strong combination': The Edwardian BMA and contract practice', in Gorsky and Sheard (eds) op. cit. (note 51), 165-81.

66. Carolyn J. Tuohy, Remaking Policy: Scale, Pace, and Political Strategy in Health Care Reform, (Toronto: University of Toronto Press, 2018).

67. John Mohan, Planning, Markets and Hospitals (London: Routledge, 2002), 181-2; Higgins, op. cit. (note 47), 85-8.

68. M. Gorsky, J. Mohan and T. Willis, 'From Hospital Contributory Schemes to Health Cash Plans: Mutualism in British Health Care after 1948', Journal of Social Policy, 34, 3 (2005), 447-67.

69. Allyson Pollock, NHS PLC: The Privatisation of Our Health Care (London: Verso Books, 2009), 60-2.

70. Enoch Powell, Speech to Annual Conference, National Association for Mental Health, 1961, cited in Jones, op cit. (note 25), 321-2.

71. Trevor Turner, 'The History of Deinstitutionalization and Reinstitutionalization', Psychiatry, 3, 9 (2004), 1-4; Peter Barham, Closing the Asylum – The Mental Patient in Modern Society (London: Penguin Books, 1992).

72. Martin Gorsky, '"To Regulate and Confirm Inequality'? A Regional History of Geriatric Hospitals under the English National Health Service, c.1948-c.1975', Ageing and Society, 33, 4 (2013), 598-625.

73. 'The Workhouse', URL http://www.workhouses.org.uk accessed 17 May 2019; Graham Moon, Robin Kearns, Alun Joseph, The Afterlives of the Psychiatric Asylum: Recycling Concepts, Sites and Memories

(Abingdon: Routledge, 2016).

74. John Appleby, 'The Hospital Bed: On its Way Out?' BMJ, 346 (2013), f1563; Leo Ewbank, James Thompson, Helen McKenna, NHS Hospital Bed Numbers: Past, Present, Future, London: Kings Fund, 2017, Figure 3, URL: https://www.kingsfund.org.uk/publications/nhs-hospital-bed-numbers accessed 19 May 2019.

75. I. Jones (ed), Health Services Financing (London: British Medical Association, 1967).

76. Lucy Reynolds and Martin McKee, 'Opening the Oyster: the 2010–11 NHS Reforms in England, Clinical Medicine, 12, 2 (2012), 128–32.

77. Higgins, op. cit. (note 47), 84-8.

78. David Turner and Thomas Powell, NHS Commissioning before April 2013, House of Commons Briefing Paper, CBP 05607, 23 September 2016.

79. Allyson Pollock and Sylvia Godden, 'Independent sector treatment centres: evidence so far', British Medical Journal, 336 (2008), 421–4; Zack Cooper, Stephen Gibbons, Matthew Skellern, 'Does Competition from Private Surgical Centres Improve Public Hospitals' Performance? Evidence from the English National Health Service', CEP Discussion Paper 1434, London: LSE, 2016.

80. A. Pollock, A. Macfarlane, G. Kirkwood, et al., 'No Evidence that Patient Choice in the NHS Saves Lives', Lancet, 378, 9809, 2057-60; Z. Cooper, S. Gibbons, S. Jones, A. McGuire, 'Does Hospital Competition Save Lives? Evidence from the NHS Patient Choice Reforms', Economic Journal, 121, 2011, 228–60.

81. Though other peer nations had similar levels to the UK: Spain (2.7), Sweden (2.7), Netherlands (2.9), see Leo Ewbank, James Thompson, Helen McKenna, NHS Hospital Bed Numbers: Past, Present, Future, London: Kings Fund, 2017, Figure 5, URL: https://www.kingsfund.org.uk/publications/nhs-hospital-bed-numbers.

82. Trevor Turner, 'Medical Milestones Chlorpromazine: unlocking psychosis', BMJ, 334 (2007), s7.

83. J. Moncrieff, The Myth of the Chemical Cure: A Critique of Psychiatric Drug Treatment (London: Palgrave Macmillan, 2008).

84. Andrew Scull, Decarceration: Community Treatment and the Deviant: a Radical View (London: Prentice-Hall, 1977).

85. David Armstrong, 'Decline of the Hospital: Reconstructing Institutional Dangers', Sociology of Health and Illness, 20 (1998), 445-7.

86. David Armstrong, 'The Rise of Surveillance Medicine', Sociology of Health and Illness, 17 (1995), 393-404.

87. David Armstrong, 'Public Health Spaces and the Fabrication of Identity', Sociology, 27 (1993), 393-410.

88. Rona Campbell, 'The Place of Birth', in Jo Alexander, Valerie Levy, Sarah Roch (eds)Intrapartum Care: A Research-Based Approach (London: Palgrave, 1990), 1-23, at 2; House of Commons Health Committee, Choice in Maternity Services. Ninth Report of Session 2002–03, Written Evidence, 'Appendix 22, Memorandum by Alison

Macfarlane and Rona Campbell'; Office of National Statistics, 'Number of live births at home and total live births, England, 1994 to 2014 birth registrations'.

89. Aneurin Bevan, In Place of Fear (London: William Heinemann, 1952), 75, 168.

90. J. Appleby, 'Government funding of the UK National Health Service: what does the historical record reveal?', Journal of Health Services Research and Policy, 4, 2 (1999), 79-89; J. Appleby '70 Years of NHS Spending', Nuffield Trust comment 2018. URL: https://www.nuffieldtrust.org.uk/news-item/70-years-of-nhs-spending.

91. Ellen Nolte, Martin McKee, 'Measuring the health of nations: analysis of mortality amenable to health care', BMJ, 327 (2003), 1129; Franco Berrino, Roberta De Angelis, Milena Sant et al., 'Survival for Eight Major Cancers and All Cancers Combined for European Adults Diagnosed in 1995-99: Results of the EUROCARE-4 study' Lancet Oncology, 8, 9 (2007), 773-783.

92. Rudolf Klein, op. cit. (note 45), 253.

93. C. Webster, The Health Services since the War, Vol. II, Government and Health Care: The National Health Service 1958–1979 (London: The Stationery Office, 1996), 822.

94. Mohan, op. cit. (note 67), 111-57.

95. P. Bridgen and J. Lewis, Elderly People and the Boundary Between Health and Social Care 1946–91 (London: Nuffield Trust, 1999).

96. M. Gorsky and G. Millward, 'Resource Allocation for Equity in the British National Health Service 1948-89: an Advocacy Coalition Analysis of the 'RAWP'', Journal of Health Policy, Politics and Law,43, 1 (2018), 69-108.

97. S. Harrison, National Health Service Management in the 1980s: Policymaking on the Hoof? (Aldershot: Avebury, 1994); M. Gorsky, "Searching for the People in Charge': Appraising the 1983 Griffiths NHS Management Inquiry', Medical History, 57, 1 (2013), 87–107.

98. Eleanor MacKillop, Sally Sheard, Philip Begley and Michael Lambert eds., The NHS Internal Market Witness Seminar (Liverpool: University of Liverpool, 2018).

99. House of Commons Health Committee, Commissioning: Fourth Report of Session 2009-10, Volume I.

100. Nick Hayes, Policy paper: Health reforms, opinion polls and surveys: myths and realities, History and Policy, 2 December 2013, Figure 2 http://www.historyandpolicy.org/policy-papers/papers/health-reforms-opinion-polls-and-surveys-myths-and-realities (accessed 13 May 2019).

101. Nicholas Timmins, Sir Michael Rawlins and John Appleby, A Terrible Beauty: A Short History of NICE (Nonthaburi: HITAP, 2016).

102. G. Bevan, M. Karanikolos, J. Exley, E. Nolte, S. Connolly and N. Mays, The four health systems of the UK: How do they compare? (London: Nuffield Trust and Health Foundation, 2014).

103. Martin Gorsky, Policy Paper: Coalition policy towards the NHS: past contexts and current trajectories, History and Policy, 3 January 2011 http://www.historyandpolicy.org/policy-papers/papers/coalition-policy-towards-the-nhs-past-contexts-and-current-trajectories (accessed 13 May 2019).

104. Chris Ham, Hugh Alderwick, Phoebe Dunn, Helen McKenna, Delivering Sustainability and Transformation Plans. From Ambitious Proposals to Credible Plans (London: Kings Fund, 2017).

105. Nick Black, 'Declining Health-Care Productivity in England: The Making of a Myth', The Lancet, 379, 9821 (2012), 1167-1169.

Chapter 6

The American Hospital: Charity, Public Service, or Profit Centre?

Beatrix Hoffman
(Northern Illinois University)

The United States has the most expensive health system in the world, costing over 17% of the country's gross national product. Of the nation's total health costs, slightly less than half is paid through the public sector (especially the programmes Medicare and Medicaid), and slightly more than half through the private sector (especially private insurance companies). The largest portion of health spending (33%) goes to hospitals, about 80% of which are designated non-profit. U.S. hospitals receive 60% of their income from taxpayer funds, and have an average profit margin of 8%. Despite its massive health expenditure, 27 million people in the U.S. have no health insurance.[1]

This brief statistical overview highlights some of the major paradoxes of the American health care and hospital systems. As Rosemary Stevens writes in her unsurpassed study *In Sickness and in Wealth*, '[t]he essential dilemma for American hospitals is that they are both public and private.'[2] The vast majority of hospitals are privately owned and operated, but receive a large part of their revenues from public spending. In addition, hospitals work both to serve the public, and to generate profits. The complex funding mechanisms and contradictory missions of U.S. hospitals have resulted in high costs and serious obstacles to universal access.

This chapter examines one particular aspect of the paradox: U.S. hospitals' obligations to serve those who cannot pay. While hospitals' commitment to the poor has changed dramatically since the nation's founding, these institutions are still expected to provide some uncompensated care, or 'charity', for the many Americans who fall through the system's gaping holes. The paradox has only intensified as hospitals partially transformed from charities to profit centres, and as funding sources moved from voluntary donations to patient fees and public and private insurance. After briefly tracing the history of these transformations, this chapter will focus on the period since 1970 to examine how the public, media, and government have responded to the tension between hospitals' profit-making and charity-giving roles. The failure of the United States to adopt universal coverage has led to the continuing practice of channeling public funds to private institutions that provide what is still called 'charity care.'

The Hospital Paradox

Hospitals in the United States fall into three general categories: voluntary (now called non-profit), public, and for-profit. The first voluntary hospitals, based on the British model of private 'non-profit institutions funded by philanthropy or patients' contributions',[3] opened in Philadelphia and New York in the two decades before the American Revolution. Public institutions run by local governments also have a long history in the U.S., including almshouses or poorhouses (which sometimes served a health care function), municipal and county hospitals, and state insane asylums. The federal (national) government funded marine hospitals for the care of sick and disabled sailors and, by the twentieth century, a system of hospitals for veterans. A third category, proprietary or for-profit hospitals, emerged in the late nineteenth century. Until the 1970s, most proprietary hospitals were small, and owned by physicians.[4]

But these categories do not capture the complex and shifting mixtures of funding sources and patient populations that characterise most hospitals in the U.S. The voluntary hospital, especially, has been a tangle of contradictions. Founded to provide free care to the indigent poor, by the late nineteenth century most had also begun accepting paying patients (in part to fund their charity services). And, although heavily dependent on individual donations, voluntary hospitals were never entirely private; state and local government contributions to these types of hospitals were common throughout the 1800s. Private charity coexisted with traditions of local government responsibility for paupers or the indigent that dated back to the Elizabethan Poor Law.[5]

Despite this long tradition of public support, voluntary hospitals vigorously asserted their autonomy from government interference, particularly their right to choose which patients to accept. This was especially true in the case of racial segregation: the widespread refusal of voluntary hospitals to accept patients of colour led to the establishment of separate institutions, owned and run by African Americans, by the late nineteenth century.[6] The ideology of voluntarism also played a powerful role in the defeat of proposals for compulsory health insurance legislation in the 1910s, when it was invoked by hospitals, physicians, and business leaders alike, who all insisted that government intervention would erode individual choice in medical care.[7]

Hospitals' mixing of public and private intensified during the Great Depression, when private voluntary hospitals insisted that they deserved increased funding from the government to meet the heavy demand from patients who could not pay. Some threatened to close their doors if state subsidies were not forthcoming. In 1934, the American Hospital Association declared that 'local government funds should be used to pay for service in voluntary hospitals' because 'the care of the indigent sick is the fundamental responsibility of government bodies.' Government responded, and by 1935, the amount received by U.S. voluntary hospitals from state and local tax funds had surpassed their receipts from private charitable giving. But the increase in government funds did not disturb the voluntary hospitals' private orientation, and indeed inspired them to reassert it. As one administrator said, hospitals should 'welcome governmental assistance to aid us in rendering help, but never permit Government to control us.'[8]

This blend of public funding and private control would find its greatest expression in the post-war federal hospital construction programme known as Hill-Burton, which emerged out of fight for national health insurance led by President Harry S. Truman from 1945 to 1950. Conservatives in Congress sought to forestall a national programme by supporting only one part of the proposal, hospital construction, that would expand access but fall far short of universal coverage. The Hill-Burton Act aimed to use federal, state, and local funds to build new hospitals in the 40% of U.S. counties that lacked them. By the end of the twentieth century, Hill-Burton would help finance 6,800 hospitals, health centres, and nursing homes in 4,000 communities around the country. Although the post-war hospital system was built with government dollars, Hill-Burton preserved hospitals' managerial autonomy by law, and even allowed Southern hospitals to continue the practice of Jim Crow racial segregation until the mid-1960s.[9]

Since Truman's national health insurance proposal was defeated, hospital construction was not accompanied by any provision for people to pay for care in the new hospitals. Hospitals themselves had already invented the Blue Cross system of service benefits for hospital care, at the beginning of the Great Depression. Throughout the 1940s and 1950s, private health insurance, including Blue Cross, Blue Shield for physicians' fees in the hospital, and commercial indemnity insurance, paid for a large and growing portion of care in hospitals (and inarguably helped encourage overuse of hospitals and subsequent inflation of hospital costs).[10] Labour unions, which had previously supported national insurance, in the 1950s decided to focus on obtaining Blue Cross or commercial hospitalisation coverage for their members through collective bargaining. This shift, alongside federal regulations that gave favorable tax status to employer-provided insurance, unintentionally created the distinctive U.S. system of health insurance tied to employment.[11]

But private health insurance left out large portions of the population: the poor, workers in jobs without benefits, and especially the elderly. Hospital and insurance officials warned that if a way was not found to cover these vulnerable groups, the government would have to step in. Their predictions came true when Medicare (social insurance coverage for people age 65 and over) and Medicaid (state-federal coverage for the poor) were approved by Congress in 1965 as part of President Lyndon B. Johnson's 'Great Society'.[12]

While bringing health coverage to millions for the first time, Medicare also proved to be a financial windfall for hospitals. Thanks to extensive lobbying by the medical profession and hospital industry, the legislation expressly forbade any regulation of physicians' fees or hospital costs. Hospitals would charge Medicare 'retrospectively' (after services were delivered) for what hospitals themselves deemed 'reasonable costs', plus an additional 2% (known as 'cost plus'). In the decade following Medicare's passage, the average cost per patient per day more than doubled, and hospitals' total assets rose from $16.4 billion to $47.3 billion. Alongside the growing costs of medical care in general (due to new technologies and treatments, higher labour costs, and overall inflation), Medicare payments to doctors and hospitals helped drive the rise in national health expenditures from $198 per capita in 1965 to $336 by 1970.[13]

The American Medical Association had hired actor Ronald Reagan in 1961 to decry the Medicare proposal as a herald of socialism.[14] But, as Rosemary Stevens has explained, Medicare's massive infusion of government funding had the ironic effect of making hospitals behave even more like private businesses. 'Market-oriented behavior,' Stevens writes, 'was a rational response by hospitals to the structures and incentives built into Medicare' that allowed hospitals to bill for whatever and how much they wished. One result of Medicare's 'golden river of money' was to 'bring hospitals into prominence as enterprises motivated by organizational self-interest, by the excitement of the game, by greed.'[15]

Medicare's largesse also encouraged for-profit hospitals to enter the game. To the nation's small sector of physician-owned proprietary hospitals were added new, massive investor-owned hospital chains, which appeared for the first time in the late 1960s directly as a result of Medicare's willingness to reimburse at cost plus— 'Essentially, the federal government gave hospitals a blank check', as business writers Sandy Lutz and E. Preston Gee put it. Copying the business model of successful hotel and fast-food chains, a new investor-owned hospital sector grew quickly. By 1971, the for-profit Hospital Corporation of America (later known as Columbia/HCA) owned 23 hospitals, and competed with 37 other investor-owned health care conglomerates.[16]

In 1980, Arnold Relman, editor of the influential *New England Journal of Medicine*, warned of a new 'medical industrial complex', 'a large and growing network of private corporations engaged in the business of supplying health-care services to patients for a profit.' Relman saw dangers in the inherent contradictions between health care as a market product and as a public good. He argued that corporate health care was at odds with the goals of cost control and improved health outcomes, because profit-making providers had no incentive to reduce utilization or to treat uninsured or very sick patients. Finally, the medical-industrial complex (as President Dwight D. Eisenhower had earlier cautioned of the military-industrial complex) could exercise 'unwarranted influence' in politics, and especially might use its new power to block regulation and comprehensive reform.[17]

Relman was certainly correct that for-profit providers would build powerful lobbying organizations and hold considerable influence over health politics.[18] But in contrasting corporate hospital chains with a non-profit sector that served as the bastion of public service and patient-oriented care, Relman's picture of the medical-industrial complex missed an even more momentous transformation: non-profit hospitals were rapidly adopting the practices of their for-profit competitors.[19]

Medicare's funding structure, as noted earlier, had already encouraged non-profits to seek ways to maximise reimbursements. As large corporate chains began to compete for patients and Medicare dollars, non-profit hospitals joined the cutthroat business game of the 1980s. Policy scholar Bradford R. Gray has noted that non-profits increasingly behaved more like for-profits throughout the decade, including moving into activities previously anathema to the charity sector like advertising and marketing, borrowing to fund capital improvements, subcontracting services, and merging and acquiring other hospitals. 'Business terminology and business thinking have pervaded the non-profit hospital world', Gray concluded in his 1991 study.[20]

One result of this increasing business orientation was a shift in hospitals' rhetoric about their role in the community. For example, Children's Memorial Hospital, a longstanding charitable institution in Chicago, issued a new mission statement in 1980 intended to 'bring Children's into the reality of the eighties.' Replacing its 1886 statement that Children's was 'dedicated exclusively to the free care and treatment of children from three to thirteen years of age', the reworded mission promised '[t]o provide infants and children the maximum quantity and quality of comprehensive health care within the available resources of the hospital.'[21]

Health writer Elisabeth Rosenthal describes a similar change of language in her description of a non-profit Catholic hospital's 'journey from charity to profit.' In the 1980s, Providence Hospital in Portland, Oregon altered its mission statement to include 'stewardship' of resources alongside more traditional religious hospital notions of justice and compassion. The Catholic nuns who ran Providence went to school for business degrees, increased the size of administration, and hired professional 'coders' to maximise Medicare billings. The hospital used borrowing and profits to invest heavily in capital 'improvements', including a lobby that welcomed patients with 'marble columns', 'a fountain with jumping salmon', and 'expensive art'. In 2013 Providence's chief executive officer was paid $3.5 million a year.[22]

In that same year, 7 of the 10 most profitable hospitals in the U.S. were 'non-profit'.[23] What, then, is the distinction between for-profit and non-profit hospitals? How have the majority (around 80%) of hospitals remained officially 'non-profit',[24] even as their profit-seeking behaviors vastly increased? In order to retain the desirable legal designation of tax-exempt charitable organizations, non-profit hospitals have had to meet certain requirements, known variously as 'charity care', 'community service', 'community benefit', and 'uncompensated care' obligations. While rooted in hospitals' charity origins, these requirements and their definitions have changed significantly over time.

Caring for the Poor: From Charitable Mission to Regulatory Requirement

'Charity' meant two somewhat different things in early U.S. hospitals. Hospitals themselves sought charitable gifts from wealthy donors and the general public to maintain buildings, pay staff, and establish endowments. At the same time, voluntary non-profit hospitals existed to *provide* charity to the deserving poor. Pennsylvania Hospital was founded in 1757 'for the relief of the sick and miserable', and its seal depicted the story of the Good Samaritan.[25] This dual charitable tradition—as receiver and giver of charity—continued even as voluntary hospitals increasingly admitted paying patients starting in the late nineteenth century.[26]

The definition of a charity hospital has never been fixed. For the nineteenth and good part of the twentieth century, hospital charitable status was based on a vague notion of 'public benefit'. As Rosemary Stevens describes it, hospitals 'did not have to offer services necessarily, or even primarily, to serve the poor... It was assumed, rather, that the act of benevolence itself...should be recognized' by charitable exemption.[27] In 1956 the Internal Revenue Service issued more specific standards for charitable hospitals, requiring them to provide 'free or reduced-care to patients unable to pay', but only within the hospital's financial ability. A little over a decade later, in 1969, the IRS eliminated this 'charity care standard' altogether, and issued a new 'community benefit standard' that allowed hospitals offering services to the community, such as an emergency room, to receive the charity designation even if they did not provide free care.[28] This change came in response to lobbying by the American Hospital Association, which had 'pushed hard for a Congressional amendment to the tax laws that would give hospitals tax exempt status' without requiring that they give free care to the poor. The Senate defeated the amendment, but it was promulgated as an IRS regulation instead, not requiring Congressional approval.[29]

Earlier, the Hill-Burton Act had created a requirement that hospitals must provide a 'reasonable volume of services' to 'persons unable to pay therefore' in order to be eligible for federal hospital construction funds. These conditions, which became known as the 'uncompensated care' and 'community service' clauses of Hill-Burton, were a nod to congressional advocates of universal access, but at the same time preserved hospitals' traditional autonomy in choosing to provide free care to those who could not pay. But the Hill-Burton Act offered no mechanism to enforce these requirements, and they went virtually ignored for two decades.

The passage of Medicare and Medicaid, alongside the surging movement for racial equality in the 1960s, led to new demands that hospitals actually meet their charity care and community service obligations. The struggle to racially integrate American hospitals had proceeded later but more swiftly than school desegregation. In 1963, a federal court ruling (*Simkins v. Cone*) declared that the Hill-Burton Act's funding of segregated hospitals violated the Fourteenth Amendment of the Constitution guaranteeing equal protection.[30] The Civil Rights Act of 1964 banned federal funding for entities that practiced discrimination, and but it was Medicare in 1965 that finally forced hospitals to stop blatant racial segregation, since hospitals found to be discriminating would be denied the new Medicare funds.[31]

Civil rights laws, however, focused entirely on *de jure* racial discrimination and did not attempt to address the poverty that disproportionately affected African Americans. Anti-poverty advocates saw greater potential in the federal-state Medicaid programme, created in 1965 alongside Medicare. Medicaid was intended to provide comprehensive health coverage to the poorest of the poor—those who were already receiving welfare (public assistance), particularly single mothers with small children. But Medicaid fell far short of universalism in two ways. First, states could decide their own eligibility requirements, and these requirements could be so stringent as to exclude many low-income people. Medicaid therefore did not eliminate the need for charity or indigent care, and in fact led to a new definition of 'indigent' as a patient too poor to pay for medical care, but ineligible for Medicaid. Second, physicians and hospitals were not required to accept patients with Medicaid (neither were they required to accept Medicare patients, but Medicaid reimbursement was far lower).[32] Because the poorest were in so many areas of the country disproportionately women of colour, hospitals' ability to refuse Medicaid patients in effect allowed them to continue to practice racial and economic discrimination.

In 1970, a landmark lawsuit in New Orleans, Louisiana challenged hospitals' refusal of low-income people. Crusading civil rights attorneys brought the suit, *Cook v. Ocshner*, as a class action on behalf of a group of poor African-American women who had been turned away from New Orleans hospitals, either because they could not pay a cash fee or because they were Medicaid recipients. The suit targeted ten hospitals that had received a total of $18 million in Hill-Burton funds. The Louisiana district court ruled that the hospitals' policy of 'sparingly admitting or refusing Medicaid patients clearly discriminated against a very substantial segment of the public and violated the 'community service' obligation under the [Hill-Burton] Act.'[33]

In response to *Cook v. Ochsner*, the federal government created new regulations in 1972 requiring Hill-Burton hospitals to devote three per cent of their operating costs to uncompensated care (the original proposal was for five per cent) and to open their doors to patients with Medicaid coverage. But would hospitals comply? Legal aid attorneys predicted that '[c]onsumers will undoubtedly still have to take an active role in enforcing the [free care and community service] requirement... after all[,] the requirement has been around for years, but the major enforcement activity came only after several lawsuits by poor consumers.'[34]

Holding Hospitals Accountable: Citizen and Government Action

Cook v. Ochsner was just the beginning of a surge of consumer and civil rights activism directed toward hospitals in the 1970s. The next section of this chapter discusses how activist groups and state and local governments responded to the growing tension between hospitals' public-service and profit-making roles by insisting that hospitals fulfill their obligations to provide some care to the poor. As Medicare, Medicaid, and Hill-Burton seemingly increased hospitals' accountability to the public and to the taxpayer, the rise of profit-seeking by hospitals (both non-profit and for-profit) brought these longstanding contradictions into even sharper relief, and new types of activism emerged in response.

Social movements—struggles for change 'from below'—have played a critical role in the United States health system. The civil rights insurgency of the 1950s and 1960s that led to sweeping legal and political changes also spurred reforms like Medicare and Medicaid, which were intended in part to bring the benefits of medical progress to the poor, elderly, and minority groups on a basis of equality. Medicare and Medicaid raised expectations that hospitals would play a role in addressing racial and economic injustices. These expectations led to citizen action that focused on hospitals' obligations to low-income Americans. In 1973 the Health Policy Advisory Committee (Health/PAC), a New Left group dedicated to health care justice, called on advocates for the poor to 'attack... private hospitals when they take public money but leave behind the public responsibility to care for everyone.'[35]

Social activism directed towards hospitals also surged in the late 1960s and 1970s because of a brief period of institutional support from a government agency, the Office of Economic Opportunity (OEO), which had begun providing legal services to anti-poverty organizations as part of Lyndon Johnson's War on Poverty.[36] OEO attorneys worked with activists from the emerging welfare rights organizations of the early 1970s to bring suits against hospitals that discriminated against the poor. This was the approach that had led to court victories in the *Cook v. Ochsner* case.

While *Cook* invoked Hill-Burton to demand that hospitals treat Medicaid and low-income patients, another legal strategy pointed to non-profit hospitals' tax-exempt status. In a 1971 case, OEO attorneys and citizens' groups in Kentucky filed a lawsuit not against individual hospitals, but against the departments of Treasury and Internal Revenue in Washington, D.C., 'for illegally granting tax exempt status as 'charitable' institutions to hospitals which refuse to treat people who can't pay.' The citizens groups involved in the suit, ranging from welfare rights and tenants' organizations to the Association of Disabled Miners and Widows, alleged that a woman died giving birth at home after the tax-exempt Prestonburg General Hospital 'refused to admit her without a $259 deposit and refused to accept a check for that deposit… The same hospital refused to treat a 5-year-old boy's broken leg because the parents had no money.'[37] By filing suit against the government rather than specific hospitals, though, the plaintiffs overreached, at least according to the U.S. Supreme Court, which ruled they had no standing to sue.[38] Later attempts to use charity tax status to demand care for the poor would focus primarily on individual hospitals (see below).

Activists also demanded strong enforcement of the new 1972 Hill-Burton uncompensated care and community service obligations. In a speech to hospital leaders, Richard H. Mapp of the Urban League, a prominent civil rights group, called the new regulations 'a minimum effort, but it was nonetheless a welcomed effort after a quarter-century of inaction.' Mapp attacked the hospital lobby's undue influence in

Washington, demanding that lawmakers 'giv[e] as much consideration to the needs and concerns of the poor as is given the hospitals and powerful medical groups who often place their own welfare above the welfare of those less fortunate than they.'[39]

But hospitals continued to find ways to evade free care requirements. In 1975 an investigation of Hill-Burton hospitals in 11 Southern states found virtually no enforcement and little provision of free care, concluding that 'it is clear that the [Hill-Burton charity care] regulations are little more than empty words...'[40] Consumer activists and advocates for the poor continued to press for stronger regulations and launched campaigns to inform patients of their rights to demand free care from hospitals. The community group Alabama Coalition Against Hunger in 1980 distributed 11,000 wallet cards to inform consumers of the Hill-Burton free care regulations. According to organisers, 'Our basic goal...was to make Hill-Burton a household word.'[41]

But Hill-Burton activists had only partial success. In 1978, 73% of hospitals in California, for example, failed to meet the free care regulations. By 1981 that number had decreased, but not by much: 45% of hospitals in the state were still out of compliance, due to 'loopholes, sloppiness and even outright lying', according to health advocates. When a 'flood of groups' including civil rights, senior citizens, and feminist health organizations testified for stronger enforcement, 'a minor furor' ensued when it was revealed that 'San Jose's O'Connor Hospital had no knowledge it was a Hill-Burton facility, despite its receipt of $1.6 million in Hill-Burton funds.'[42] That a hospital itself was unaware of its obligations and its funding source, despite activists' attempt to make Hill-Burton a 'household word', points to the daunting complexity of U.S. hospital financing and its byzantine regulatory regime—obstacles not only to enforcement, but to basic public understandings of how hospitals function, and corresponding difficulties for social movements to effect change.[43]

In the budget-cutting frenzy of the 1980s, the Reagan administration reduced Medicaid reimbursements so severely that hospitals drastically increased 'patient dumping', the practice of transferring uninsured or Medicaid patients from private to public hospitals. In 1984 the city of Chicago experienced a 500% increase in such transfers, from less than 100 to 600-700 a month.[44] Dumping became so widespread that in 1986 Congress created the Emergency Medical Treatment and Active Labor Act (EMTALA), requiring hospitals to examine and stabilise all patients who arrived at the emergency room. While EMTALA reduced but did not completely end the practice of patient dumping, the law cemented the emergency room's role as the only place in the U.S. health care system where access is legally required. EMTALA did not create a new obligation to provide free care; it only requires hospitals to wait to bill patients until after they are stabilised. Since it also tended to increase costs by encouraging expensive emergency room visits, EMTALA was not seen as a victory by health justice advocates.[45]

In the 1980s and 1990s, hospital activists confronted the growing power of the for-profit sector as private corporations like Columbia/ Hospital Corporation of America (HCA) acquired hospital systems throughout the country. In Houston, Texas, for example, for-profit giant Humana operated three hospitals, eight clinics, and the group health insurance plan and HMO (Health Maintenance Organization) that financed patient care in all its facilities. This health-care consolidation, reminiscent of the age of Rockefeller, came under criticism by local physicians (and the Health/PAC advocacy organization, which referred to the situation as 'Humana-izing Health Care'). In response, Humana agreed to lease out management of the clinics, but retained control over its hospitals and health insurance plans.[46]

Advocates feared that the growing power of for-profit hospital corporations would lead to further abrogation of hospitals' responsibilities to the poor. In Kentucky, Humana's corporate home state, the firm owned seven hospitals but refused to pay into a state 'Fair Share' fund to 'spread the burden of caring for the uninsured.' Humana insisted that it contributed to care of the poor 'by paying taxes on the money it makes, and by treating indigents at [Louisville's] University Hospital.' Indeed, Humana paid the state $6 million annually to rent the formerly non-profit University Hospital. But a newspaper investigation found that almost the entire $6 million actually went right back to Humana in the form of state payments for indigent care. Humana Chairman David A. Jones defended his company's practices, stating that '[i]ndigent care is a societal problem that must be solved by government, not the hospital industry.' The Louisville *Courier-Journal* pointed out that Humana earned $193 million in profits in 1984 and paid Jones $18.1 million, making him the second-highest paid executive in the country.[47]

Humana would eventually sell its hospitals and move into the more lucrative health insurance business, but its rival Columbia/HCA soon took its place as the for-profit nemesis of the consumer movement. By the mid-90s Columbia/HCA owned 350 hospitals throughout the country and took in $20 billion in revenues. As the chain continued to aggressively pursue new acquisitions, some communities began to push back. Rhode Island's attorney general cancelled Columbia/HCA's attempted 1997 purchase of a non-profit hospital after protests by senior citizens and nurses' organizations and an investigation by state representative Patrick J. Kennedy (son of Edward Kennedy and nephew of JFK).[48]

When advocates failed to prevent for-profit acquisitions, they demanded promises of continued charity obligations from the new owners. In the late 1990s HCA/Columbia acquired two major nonprofit hospitals in San Jose, California and proposed merging them. Consumer groups sought a commitment to 'more free medical care for San Jose residents as part of the hospital transfer.'[49] When two for-profit giants

(Vanguard and Tenet) vied to purchase non-profit Allegheny Health Network's bankrupt chain of Philadelphia hospitals in 1998, protesters under the banner of 'Coalition for Patients Not Profits' declared 'We must send a loud and clear message to the new owner of Allegheny that we intend to protect our indigent poor.' The Coalition, which included senior citizens, welfare rights, and provider groups, demanded that the new owners not close hospitals or reduce service and 'maintain an obligation to provide care for the indigent.'[50]

Absent Hill-Burton funding and tax exemptions, for-profit hospitals had no official or enforceable requirements to provide care to the uninsured (except for emergency care). When for-profits entered hospital markets, activists and local governments tried to extract guarantees of commitment to the poor via ad hoc agreements and simple promises. Such arrangements were even more difficult to enforce than the anemic Hill-Burton and IRS requirements. As with non-profits, some for-profit hospitals provided a notable amount of free care, some (like Humana) very little (exact amount are impossible to measure due to, of course, little to no enforcement and scattershot reporting requirements).[51] In the new millennium, debates over the for-profit sector's contribution to charity care faded as public attention turned to new scandals. In 2000, Columbia/HCA paid $95 million to settle multiple accusations of fraud, which included massively overbilling Medicare and providing financial rewards to physicians who referred patients to HCA hospitals. Leaders of HealthSouth Corporation, which owned rehabilitation hospitals and clinics throughout the U.S. South, actually went to prison in 2006 for accounting fraud and bribery.[52]

Despite their aggressive acquisitions and high-profile antics, for-profit hospitals did not come to dominate the U.S. health system. After many selloffs, and with some big players (such as Humana) abandoning the industry altogether, today for-profits constitute only about 25% of all community hospitals.[53] The tension between hospitals' charity and profit missions would reach a boiling point not in the for-profit sector, but the non-profit, as the revenue-maximizing behavior of an esteemed academic medical centre led to a public outcry.

The scandal involved the Yale-New Haven Medical System in Connecticut, which included Yale University's storied hospital and medical college as well as other non-profit hospitals around the state. In the 1990s, Yale-New Haven adopted new, aggressive collections tactics to recoup money owed by former patients. These practices became national news when the *Wall Street Journal* reported the story of a 77-year old New Haven man who still owed the hospital tens of thousands of dollars for his late wife's cancer treatment. Yale-New Haven 'sued him, put a lien on his house and seized most of his bank account.'[54] The hospital system took uninsured former patients to court, garnished up to 25% of their paychecks, and even forced them to foreclose on their homes. Connecticut labour unions and anti-poverty advocates who publicised these stories emphasised how Yale-New Haven's harsh tactics stood in sharp relief against its status as 'a non-profit, charitable teaching hospital…the largest, most prestigious hospital in the state and the largest 'safety-net' provider of healthcare to the poor and uninsured in the city of New Haven.'[55]

The publicity led to protests that were 'long, loud, and visible.' A health care workers union erected a large billboard, that could be seen from the main hospital's windows, containing only the word 'SHAME.' The state attorney general and lawmakers stepped in, and soon the hospital system changed its billing practices and, in 2005, replaced its entire leadership. Today, Yale-New Haven has become a model of cooperation with the local community, including providing funding for clinics and donating land for low-income housing.[56]

But the lessons of Yale's scandal did not change much behavior in the non-profit hospital sector. Throughout the 2000s, non-profits' profit-seeking, charity-minimizing actions continued to elicit shock from the public, media, and local politicians. For example, a 2005 investigation by the *Salt Lake Tribune* found that the Intermountain Hospital Corporation (IHC), which operated 19 hospitals and numerous clinics in the state of Utah, filed 723 debt-collection lawsuits in a single year. Intermountain, which included the University of Utah hospital, was a fully non-profit chain. 'Charities shouldn't sue people', health activist Steven DeVore told the *Tribune*. DeVore lobbied unsuccessfully for state legislators to revoke IHC's tax-exempt status.[57]

To counter arguments like DeVore's, non-profits frequently, and ironically, justified their aggressive billing practices by invoking their status as charity institutions. They had to pursue every possible dollar to cover the costs of free care, they argued.'[W]e provide a lot of charity, and do a lot of good in the community', an Ohio hospital executive told National Public Radio. In order to provide that charity, 'we have to collect payment from those who can afford to pay us.'[58]

The non-charitable behaviors of non-profit hospitals brought further attention to the question of tax exemption. In the most well-known example, tax officials in Champaign, Illinois revoked the tax-exempt status of Provena Hospital in 2003 for failing to provide sufficient charity care. Provena was a Catholic hospital, but its $800,000 annual expenditure on 'charitable activities' was less than its $1.1 million savings in local property taxes. Even though neither federal nor Illinois law specified how much charity care or community benefit non-profits were required to provide to maintain their status, the state Supreme Court agreed that Provena no longer qualified as a charity. The Illinois Hospital Association, the state lobbying group for the hospitals, objected to the decision on the grounds that 'Imposing new tax burdens on a hospital could force it to reduce services and increase health care costs.'[59]

The growing attention to hospitals' behavior from activists, media, and state governments was not welcomed, but could no longer be ignored. What one reporter called the 'uninsured billing/charity-care tsunami' (meaning the flood of bad publicity for hospitals) was leading to a moment of reckoning. 'There is no question', the industry journal *Modern Healthcare* admitted in 2004, 'that a lack of clarity of mission and poor reporting by many in the industry invited this deluge of scrutiny...Some hospitals and systems really do act like for-profits, and they threaten to damage the many providers with a patient-first mentality.'[60] More unwelcome publicity arrived in the form of a series of class action lawsuits brought by high-profile anti-tobacco attorney Richard Scruggs against twelve hospital systems across the country. The suits alleged that the hospitals 'failed to conduct [themselves] as the charitable entit[ies they] purport to be', that they provided insufficient care to the poor and uninsured, and that they 'charged unreasonable and excessive rates for medical care' and engaged in 'aggressive, abusive and humiliating collections practices.' The *Wall Street Journal* noted that 'The suits are coming at a difficult juncture for the hospital industry, whose practices toward the uninsured are under scrutiny.'[61]

Scruggs's class action lawsuits failed; judges ruled that only the government, not private individuals in court actions, could enforce the tax code against hospitals.[62] Still, the industry had been put on the defensive. If hospitals did not take steps to show they were deserving of their tax exemptions, *Modern Healthcare* warned, government would step in.[63]

This prediction came true in 2006 when a Congressional sub-committee began investigating non-profit hospital practices, and the *New York Times* reported that Congress 'will set standards for the industry if it does not do so itself.'[64] Iowa Senator Charles Grassley, a longtime critic of the hospital industry, was angered that hospitals 'continu[ed] to act uncharitably'; not only did they fail to provide significant charity care, but they also paid excessively high salaries to executives, and used their profits to move out of poor areas and build new hospitals in wealthier suburbs. Grassley wanted to impose minimum requirements for uncompensated care, and to fine hospitals that did not comply.[65] He would soon have an opportunity to bring his proposals to fruition, as Congress enacted, and Barack Obama signed into law, the most sweeping changes to the health system since Medicare and Medicaid.

The Affordable Care Act and the Fate of Charity Care

In 2010, Congress passed the Patient Protection and Affordable Care Act, the most far-reaching health reform since Medicare. The legislation, which became known as the Affordable Care Act (ACA) or Obamacare, represented a retreat from the goal of universal coverage that health reformers had sought for decades. Instead, the ACA attempted to expand health coverage incrementally, by expanding Medicaid and creating a system of subsidised private insurance plans.[66] Since the Supreme Court in 2012 made Medicaid expansion voluntary on the part of the states, the ACA ended up covering even fewer people than expected. Although Obamacare has extended health protection to around 20 million people, over 25 million Americans remained uninsured at the end of 2018.[67] The need for 'indigent care' is far from over.

The drafters of the ACA assumed that charity care by hospitals needed to continue, but that it would be balanced out by new benefits to hospitals. They argued that hospitals that treated large numbers of uninsured people would receive a vast increase in reimbursements from the coverage expansions. In exchange for the projected billions of dollars in new patient revenues (and to help fund the new system), the ACA would implement cuts to Medicare reimbursements and subsidies, and require greater safety and quality accountability from hospitals. As one medical journal put it, the ACA 'both giveth to and taketh away from hospitals.'[68]

This was also true in the case of charity care. The ACA, especially through the Medicaid expansion, explicitly intended to reduce the volume of uncompensated care hospitals were expected to carry. But non-profit hospitals also faced stronger reporting requirements to maintain their charitable tax status. The ACA requires hospitals to file new reports with the IRS enumerating 'how much money-losing care they dispense—and how they calculate that number. They also have to list and value what they've done gratis to better their communities.'[69] Other provisions reflected Sen. Grassley's and patient advocates' earlier criticisms of non-profit hospital practices by banning non-profit hospitals from taking 'extreme collections actions' and charging higher rates to uninsured patients.[70]

Rather than heralding a new era in hospital accountability, the ACA charity care rules are more a case of things remaining the same. They set requirements for reporting, but not a requirement for actual amounts of charity care required. Hospitals can still define charity care as they wish, reporting a wide variety of activities as 'uncompensated care.' And they can even opt out of free care completely by paying a $50,000 fine—a tiny portion of hospital revenues. At least one hospital has in fact lost its tax exempt status since implementation of the ACA, but the new charity care mandates are, according to a trade newsletter, 'perhaps too vague to be effective.'[71]

It's not surprising that the Affordable Care Act reflects the contradictory and ambivalent roles of hospitals in the U.S. health system. Its attempt to reinforce hospitals' commitment to uncompensated care seemingly contradicts the ACA's overall goal of reducing the need for uncompensated care altogether. Following the Act's implementation in 2004, the amount of uncompensated care provided by hospitals did indeed decline, from a peak of $46.4 billion in 2013to $42.8 billion in 2014, and to $35.7 billion in 2015.[72] In states that did expand Medicaid, hospitals experienced significant reductions in charity care. At Seattle's Harborview Medical Center, for example, the proportion of uninsured patients fell from 12% in 2013 to an 'unprecedented' low of 2% in 2014.[73]

But as the Affordable Care Act faced both judicial challenge and repeated attempts at repeal by a Republican-majority Congress, it became clear that the need for uncompensated care would continue and perhaps even rise. The greatest blow to the ACA's success has been the Supreme Court 2012 ruling in *NFIB v. Sebelius* that upheld the Act but struck down its requirement that all states expand their Medicaid programmes for the poor. As of January 2019, 14 conservative-run states have refused the federal government's offer of billions of dollars in Medicaid subsidies to cover low-income working people. Only those states that accepted Medicaid expansion have seen a significant drop in the demand for charity care.

In addition, many of the newly-insured under the ACA have purchased the lowest-cost subsidised plans, which include extremely high cost-sharing in the form of deductibles and co-payments. By 2016, it was becoming evident that increasing numbers of patients with high-deductible policies were leading to more unpaid debts to hospitals.[74] Finally, there continues to be millions of uninsured people. These shortfalls in coverage have led hospital organisations to ask for increased funding for uncompensated care. The trade journal *Modern Healthcare* called for 'the next Congress [to] reconsider the assumption in the ACA that uncompensated care for the poor and uninsured would begin to fade away. As long as exchange enrollment lags and many states refuse to expand Medicaid, the nation's safety net hospitals will need—and deserve—additional support.'[75]

In seeking more taxpayer funding even as they continue to behave like private businesses, hospitals are continuing a strategy that is over a century old. American hospitals, with their powerful lobbying organizations, have proven adept at having their cake and eating it too—maximizing their profits while depending on significant subsidies from government. Despite its intentions, the Affordable Care Act has not disrupted the United States's reliance on heavily subsidised private voluntarism to compensate for the nation's refusal to adopt universal, comprehensive coverage. Like Medicare before it, the ACA preserved and reinforced the hospital's dual role as both charity and profit centre, rather than a public service available on equal terms to all.

1. Centers for Medicare and Medicaid Services, 'National Health Expenditures 2017 Highlights', https://www.cms.gov/Research-Statistics-Data-and-Systems/Statistics-Trends-and-Reports/NationalHealthExpendData/downloads/highlights.pdf; Kaiser Health News, 'Government now pays for nearly 50% of health care spending', KHN Morning Briefing, 21 February 2019, https://khn.org/morning-breakout/government-now-pays-for-nearly-50-percent-of-health-care-spending-an-increase-driven-by-baby-boomers-shifting-into-medicare/; Kaiser Family Foundation, 'Key Facts about the Uninsured Population', 7 December 2018, https://www.kff.org/uninsured/fact-sheet/key-facts-about-the-uninsured-population/; David Belk MD, 'True Cost of Health-care' Hospital Financial Analysis, http://truecostofhealthcare.org/aha-records/.

2. Rosemary Stevens, In Sickness and in Wealth: American Hospitals in the Twentieth Century (New York: Basic Books, 1989).

3. Martin Gorsky, John Mohan, and Martin Powell, 'The financial health of voluntary hospitals in interwar Britain', Economic History Review Vol. 55, 3, August (2002), 533-57 (quote on 533).

4. On nineteenth-century hospitals, see Charles Rosenberg, The Care of Strangers: The Rise of America's Hospital System (New York: Basic, 1987); Guenter B. Risse, Mending Bodies, Saving Souls: A History of Hospitals (New York: Oxford University Press, 1999).

5. Rosemary Stevens, "A Poor Sort of Memory': Voluntary Hospitals and Government Before the Great Depression', Milbank Memorial Fund Quarterly Health and Society, Vol., 60, No. 4, 1982, 551-584.

6. On hospital segregation, see, e.g., Vanessa Northington Gamble, Making a Place for Ourselves: The Black Hospital Movement, 1920-1945 (New York: Oxford, 1995); Samuel Kelton Roberts, Infectious Fear: Politics, Disease, and the Health Effects of Segregation (Chapel Hill: UNC Press, 2009).

7. Ronald Numbers, Almost Persuaded: American Physicians and Compulsory Health Insurance, 1912-1920 (Baltimore: Johns Hopkins, 1978); Beatrix Hoffman, The Wages of Sickness: The Politics of Health Insurance in Progressive America (Chapel Hill: UNC Press, 2001).

8. Beatrix Hoffman, Health Care for Some: Rights and Rationing in the United States since 1930 (Chicago: University of Chicago Press), 68.

9. On the Jim Crow hospital system, see David Barton Smith, Health Care Divided: Race and Healing a Nation (Ann Arbor: University of Michigan Press, 1999); Karen Kruse Thomas, Deluxe Jim Crow: Civil Rights and American Health Policy (Athens: University of Georgia Press, 2011).

10. Robert Cunningham III and Robert M. Cunningham, Jr., The Blues: A History of the Blue Cross Blue Shield System (DeKalb: Northern Illinois University Press, 1997).

11. On labour's role in the rise of the private insurance system, see Christy Ford Chapin, Ensuring America's Health: The Public Creation of the Corporate Health Care System (New York: Cambridge University Press,

2015); Jennifer Klein, For All These Rights: Business, Labor, and the Shaping of America's Public-Private Welfare State (Princeton: Princeton University Press, 2003).

12. After the failure of national health insurance in 1950, reformers pushed for insurance to cover the elderly only, which became known as Medicare. Existing programmes providing federal subsidies for the very poor were consolidated and attached to the 1965 Medicare bill under the new name 'Medicaid.' See, e.g., Alan B. Cohen, David C. Colby, Keith A. Wailoo, and Julian E. Zelizer, eds., Medicare and Medicaid at 50: America's Entitlement Programs in the Age of Affordable Care (New York: Oxford, 2015).

13. Centers for Medicare and Medicaid Services, National Health Expenditure Accounts https://www.cms.gov/Research-Statistics-Data-and-Systems/Statistics-Trends-and-Reports/NationalHealthExpendData/NationalHealthAccountsHistorical.html.

14. American Medical Association Communications Division, 'Ronald Reagan Speaks Out Against Socialized Medicine', audio recording, 1962.

15. Rosemary Stevens, The Public-Private Health Care State (New Brunswick, N.J.: Transaction Press, 2007), 311, 319.

16. Sandy Lutz and E. Preston Gee, The For-Profit Healthcare Revolution: The Growing Impact of Investor-Owned Health Systems (Chicago, Ill: Irwin Professional, 1995), 9-11.

17. Arnold S. Relman, M.D., 'The New Medical Industrial Complex', New England Journal of Medicine, 303 (23 October 1980), 963-970.

18. The for-profit health industry's lobbying groups include the Federation of American Hospitals and America's Health Insurance Plans. For a discussion of their influence on the Affordable Care Act, for example, see John F. McDonough, Inside National Health Reform (Berkeley: University of California Press, 2011).

19. In this way, non-profit hospitals mimicked their insurance industry counterpart, Blue Cross Blue Shield, which in the 1970s had begun to adopt commercial insurance practices in order to remain competitive. By 1994, the Blue Cross Blue Shield Association began allowing its plans to convert to for-profit. Cunningham and Cunningham, The Blues; Deborah Stone, 'The Struggle for the Soul of Health Insurance', Journal of Health Politics, Policy, and Law (1993) 18 (2), 287-317.

20. Bradford H. Gray, The Profit Motive and Patient Care: The Changing Accountability of Doctors and Hospitals (Cambridge, Mass.: Harvard University Press, 1991), 67. As much as non-profits were forced into a competitive posture by for-profit growth, the ideological environment of the 1980s (Reaganism, the cultural glorification of ruthless business practices) may also have played a role; further research is needed to weigh the material and ideological motivations of hospital leadership during this time.

21. Clare McCausland, An Element of Love: A History of the Children's Memorial Hos-

pital of Chicago, Illinois (Chicago: The Hospital, 1981), 192.

22. Elisabeth Rosenthal, An American Sickness: How Healthcare Became Big Business and How You Can Take It Back (New York: Penguin, 2017), 24-28.

23. Ge Bai and Gerard F. Anderson, 'A More Detailed Understanding of Factors Associated With Hospital Profitability', Health Affairs, Vol. 35, No. 5, 889-97.

24. American Hospital Association, Fast Facts on U.S. Hospitals, 2019 https://www.aha.org/statistics/fast-facts-us-hospitals.

25. 'History of Pennsylvania Hospital', http://www.uphs.upenn.edu/paharc/timeline/1751/. The undeserving and undesirable were the purview of government hospitals and asylums; Stevens, In Sickness and in Wealth, 27.

26. On the increased reliance on paying patients, see David Rosner, A Once Charitable Enterprise: Hospitals and Health Care in Brooklyn and New York, 1885-1915 (New York: Cambridge University Press, 1982).

27. Stevens, "A Poor Sort of Memory', 555-58; Stevens, In Sickness and in Wealth, 41. See also Internal Revenue Service, 'The Concept of Charity' (1980), https://www.irs.gov/pub/irs-tege/eotopicb80.pdf.

28. Congressional Research Service, '503(c)(3) Hospitals and the Community Benefit Standard', https://www.everycrsreport.com/reports/RL34605.html. In 2011 the tax benefit to non-profit hospitals as was estimated to be $24.6 billion.

29. 'Hospitals and Taxes', Health Law Newsletter, Issue No. 4, August 1971, 1.

30. See for example Smith, Health Care Divided. Simkins was upheld (but not decided) by the U.S. Supreme Court.

31. Jill Quadagno, One Nation, Uninsured (New York: Oxford University Press, 2006); David Barton Smith, The Power to Heal: Civil Rights, Medicare, and the Struggle to Transform America's Health Care System (Nashville: Vanderbilt University Press, 2016).

32. On Medicaid, see Jamila Michener, Fragmented Democracy: Medicaid, Federalism, and Unequal Politics (New York: Cambridge University Press, 2018) and the classic, Robert Stevens and Rosemary Stevens, Welfare Medicine in America: A Case Study of Medicaid (New York: Free Press, 1974).

33. Cook v. Ochsner Foundation Hospital, 319 F. Supp. 603 (E.D. Louisiana 1970); Beatrix Hoffman, 'Don't Scream Alone: The Health Care Activism of Poor Americans in the 1970s', in B. Hoffman, Nancy Tomes, Rachel Grob, and Mark Schlesinger, eds., Patients as Policy Actors (New Brunswick: Rutgers University Press, 2011).

34. Marilyn G. Rose, 'Federal Regulation of Services to the Poor under the Hill-Burton Act: Realities and Pitfalls', Northwestern Law Review Vol. 70, No. 1 (1975): 168-201; 'Hill-Burton', Health Law Newsletter, Issue No. 13, May 1972, 1.

35. 'Turning Point for Public Hospitals', Health/PAC Bulletin, Vol. 51, April 1973, 3.

36. On the role of 'poverty lawyers', see Martha F. Davis, Brutal Need: Lawyers and the Welfare Rights Movement, 1960-1973 (New Haven: Yale University Press, 1993); on the U.S. welfare rights movement generally, see, e.g., Annelise Orleck, Storming Caesar's Palace: How Black Women Fought Their Own War on Poverty (New York: Penguin, 2005).

37. 'Hospitals and Taxes', Health Law Newsletter, Issue No. 4, August 1971, 1.

38. Simon v. Eastern Kentucky Welfare Rights Organization (1976), https://www.law.cornell.edu/supremecourt/text/426/26.

39. Press release n.d. ca 1979, Leadership Council on Civil Rights II, Box 41, Folder 10, Manuscript Division, Library of Congress; Richard H. Mapp of National Urban League statement to Federal Hospital Council, Oct. 20, 1972. LCCR I: 129.

40. 'South's hospitals fail to meet free care rules, council says', Hospitals, March 1, 1975, Vol. 49, 118-119. The report was by the Southern Regional Council, a civil rights group.

41. Alan Seltzer and Armin Freifeld to Hill-Burton Advocates, 14 June 1979, LCCRII, Box 41, Folder 6, Library of Congress; 'Ups and Downs of Hill-Burton', Health Law Newsletter, No. 106, February 1980; 'Trainings Pay Off, Bring Increased Advocacy', NHeLP Health Advocate, No. 111, August 1980.

42. 'Tougher Hill-Burton Regs Demanded in California', NHeLP Health Advocate, No. 124, Sept. 1981, 4.

43. For a more detailed examination of how the complexity of the US health care system has fragmented social movement efforts for reform, see Beatrix Hoffman, 'Health Care Reform and Social Movements in the United States', American Journal of Public Health, 93, 1 (January 2003): 75–85.

44. Sally Guttmacher, 'Poor People, Poor Care', Health/PAC Bulletin Vol. 15, No., 4, July-August 1984, 15.

45. Beatrix Hoffman, 'Emergency Rooms: The Reluctant Safety Net', in Rosemary A. Stevens, Charles E. Rosenberg, and Lawton R. Burns, eds., History and Health Policy in the United States: Putting the Past Back In (New Brunswick: Rutgers University Press, 2006).

46.'Humana-izing Health Care', Health/PAC Bulletin Vol 16 No. 2, March-April 1985, 6. Health Maintenance Organizations, officially recognised by Congress in 1973, are insurance plans that allow members to use only a limited network of doctors and hospitals in order to reduce costs. On the early history of HMOs, see Klein, For All These Rights; on their later development, see, e.g., Bradford H. Gray, 'The Rise and Decline of the HMO: A Chapter in US Health-Policy History', in Stevens et. al. History and Health Policy in the United States.

47. 'Dynamic firm is major force, but its power worries some', Louisville Courier-Journal, 5 May 1985; 'Trial marriage with U of L has resulted in both spats and successes', Courier-Journal, 9 May 1985; 'Hospital finances now sound, but fund for poor is assailed', unidentified clipping; Jones salary, Modern Healthcare, 10 May 1985; all clippings in Papers of John R. Mannix, Box 170, File 4

'Humana', American Hospital Association Resource Center.

48. Martin Gottlieb and Kurt Eichenwald, 'A hospital chain's brass knuckles, and the backlash', New York Times, 11 May 1997.

49. Lisa M. Krieger, 'San Jose, Calif., Groups Protest Hospital Consolidation Plans', San Jose Mercury News, 30 April 30, 1999 (Newspaper Source database).

50. Karl Stark, 'Philadelphia Consumers Group Protests Proposed Sale of Allegheny Hospitals', The Philadelphia Inquirer, 5 May 1998; Andrea Ahles, 'Advocacy Group Protests Sale of Philadelphia Hospitals to For-Profit Company', The Philadelphia Inquirer, 20 August 1998 (Newspaper Source). On the Allegheny bankruptcy, see Lawton R. Burns and Alexandra P. Burns, 'Policy Implications of Hospital System Failures: The Allegheny Bankruptcy', in Stevens et. al. History and Health Policy in the United States.

51. In 2011, 15 states had charity care requirements for hospital tax exemption and/or expansion. In Atlanta between 2006-09, some for-profit hospitals provided more charity care than the city's non-profit Piedmont Hospital, which spent less than 3% of its gross income on uncompensated care. https://www.ajc.com/news/local/charity-care-hospital-regulations-scrutinized/KmeCPOUalGN5pAYS4iCyeO/

52. On the Columbia/HCA scandal, see Kurt Eichenwald, 'HCA to pay $95 million in fraud case', New York Times, 15 December 2005. Rick Scott, later Governor of Florida and now U.S. Senator, was head of Columbia/HCA during much of the scandal. On HealthSouth, see David McCann, 'Two CEOs Tell a Tale of Fraud at HealthSouth', CFO, 27 March 2017, http://www.cfo.com/fraud/2017/03/two-cfos-tell-tale-fraud-healthsouth/.

53. American Hospital Association, 'Fast Facts on U.S. Hospitals', 2019 https://www.aha.org/statistics/fast-facts-us-hospitals.

54. Dan Diamond, 'A tarnished hospital tries to win back trust', Politico, 31 December 2017, https://www.politico.com/story/2017/12/31/yale-new-haven-hospital-community-trust-261660.

55. Connecticut Center for a New Economy, 'Uncharitable Care: Yale-New Haven Hospital's Charity Care and Collections Practices'.

56. Diamond, 'A tarnished hospital'.

57. Linda Fantin, 'Salt Lake City residents say hospitals have harassed them over unpaid bills', Salt Lake Tribune, 1 October 2005.

58. Jenny Gold, 'Nonprofit hospitals faulted for stinginess with charity care', All Things Considered, 27 April 2012, https://www.npr.org/sections/health-shots/2012/04/27/151537743/nonprofit-hospitals-faulted-for-stinginess-with-charity-care. Hospitals and insurance companies often defend their high costs as the result of cost shifting and cross-subsidization required by a fragmented health system, but this can be more of a rhetorical strategy than an economic reality. See e.g., Austin B. Frakt, 'How much do hospitals cost shift? A review of the evidence', Milbank Quarterly, 89, 1 (March 2011): 90–130.

59. Lorene Yue and Mike Colias, 'Illinois Supreme Court upholds ruling against Provena in tax-exempt case', Crain's Chicago Business, 18 March 2010.

60. Todd Sloane op ed, Modern Healthcare, 5 July 2004, Vol. 34 Issue 27, 17.

61. Order by Joan Gottschall, District Judge, Watts v. Advocate Health Care Network, U.S. District Court, N.D. Illinois, Eastern Division, 30 March 2005, https://www.casemine.com/judgement/us/5914754cadd-7b049343adff6. 'Lawsuits Challenge Charity Hospitals on Care for Uninsured', Wall Street Journal, 17 June 2004: B.1.

62. Gottschall order. See also Robert Pear, 'Nonprofit hospitals face scrutiny over practices', New York Times, 19 March 2006, 18.

63. Sloane op ed, Modern Healthcare.

64. Pear, 'Nonprofit hospitals face scrutiny'.

65. John Carreyou and Barbara Martinez, 'Grassley targets nonprofit hospitals on charity care', Wall Street Journal, 18 December 2008, A5.

66. On the politics shaping the Affordable Care Act, see McDonough, Inside National Health Reform.

67. Kaiser Family Foundation, 'Key Facts about the Uninsured', December 2018, https://www.kff.org/uninsured/factsheet/key-facts-about-the-uninsured-population/

68. Andrew M. Ryan and Alvin I. Mushlin, 'The Affordable Care Act's Payment Reforms and the Future of Hospitals', Annals of Internal Medicine 160, 10 (2014), 729-730.

69. Rosenthal, An American Sickness, 50. The new IRS form is Schedule H, Form 990.

70. Beckers' Hospital Review, https://www.beckershospitalreview.com/finance/health-reforms-new-charity-care-requirements-for-hospitals-achieving-compliance-to-avoid-penalities.html

71. https://www.beckershospitalreview.com/finance/irs-revokes-hospital-s-tax-exempt-status-for-failure-to-comply-with-aca-rule.html; Jacqueline DiChiara, 'The Affordable Care Act's Effect on Hospital Charity Care', Revcycle Intelligence, 10 February 2016 https://revcycleintelligence.com/news/the-affordable-care-acts-effect-on-hospital-charity-care.

72. Tara Bannow, 'Hospital profits, uncompensated care climb', Modern Healthcare, 8 Jan. 2018, Vol. 48 Issue 2.

73. Phil Galewitz, 'An Obamacare winner: safety-net hospitals', USA Today, 24 May 2014.'The share of uninsured patients was cut roughly in half this year at two other major safety net hospitals—Denver Health in Colorado and the University of Arkansas for Medical Sciences Hospital (UAMS) in Little Rock.'

74. Scott Gottlieb, 'ObamaCare may be growing the number of unpaid medical bills', Forbes, 19 February 2016.

75. Merrill Goozner, 'An unfair DSH formula for safety net hospitals', Modern Healthcare, 11 July 2016, Vol. 46 Issue 27.

Chapter 7

The rise of hospital centrism in China, 1835-2018, from the perspective of financing[1]

Jin Xu
(Peking University)

Anne Mills
(London School of Hygiene & Tropical Medicine)

Introduction

China was once considered an international model for low cost rural primary health care. Its historical achievement in improving health at very low cost provided some of the strongest empirical evidence supporting the World Health Organization's 1978 Declaration on Primary Health Care.[2] However, over recent decades the country has suffered from an over-concentration of high-quality resources in hospitals, despite efforts to strengthen primary care.[3] In this essay we examine the reasons for this apparently contradictory situation.

Our focus is on the historical evolution of hospitals and primary care in China from the perspective of financing, drawing from a historical study covering the years 1835 to 2018. 1835 is the starting point, as it marked the founding of the first Western medical institution in China. As we have argued elsewhere, this was the inception of a hospital-centric health system model.[4] We end in 2018 in order to link the historical analysis to the contemporary situation, in which hospital-centrism remains. Two other milestones, 1949 and 1978, represent key intermediate points: in 1949, the new People's Republic of China was founded, leading China towards rapid industrialization; and 1978 marked the start of the systematic reform that shifted China's economy away from command and control and towards the market.

We begin by showing that foreign actors, whose concern was not to achieve broad health service coverage, introduced the hospital-centric model. This model was unaffordable given China's lack of industrialisation before 1949 and it remained partially unaffordable between 1949 and 1978. Hospitals in China had a high-cost orientation that was excessive for the rural population. Hence, when the country's leaders attempted to extend health services to the whole population, they faced enormous challenges in finding sufficient financial resources, and repeatedly pushed towards a lower-cost model built around primary care. The result was a divided structure. As industrialisation rapidly progressed and fiscal space expanded after 1978, wider coverage became not only feasible but also politically important, particularly after 2002. However, efforts to reorient the health system towards primary care faced a complex set of challenges, which along with the policy choices made since 1978, affected primary care strengthening.

Our conceptual approach draws particularly on two strands in the historiography of the welfare state, historical institutionalism and transnational diffusion. Much of the literature explaining the rise and development of welfare and health systems has been Western-focused, so we have approached it selectively to find a helpful lens to view the situation in China. The early structural-functionalist analysis treated welfare states as general processes arising from industrialisation, a response to market failures in the social realm. Others paid more attention to the interaction of social forces in the political arena.

The Marxist tradition emphasised class conflict and the concern of the labour movement to orient state power away from capitalist priorities. Pluralist approaches focused on other types of economic or professional vested interests, treating the democratic state as a neutral presence responding to external social actors.[5] These interpretations, however, have been found inadequate to explain the timings and configurations of national welfare states in health and in general,[6] and thus do not fit well our attention to the historical evolution of hospitals and primary care in China.

Historical-institutionalists have instead focused on the state as an autonomous force. Some emphasise the agency of state bureaucrats as key actors with varied capacities, who are not just strictly executing the interests of certain social groups, or obediently answering the call of ideologies, but leading the development of policies.[7] Others have focused on the ways in which constitutional arrangements for governing and law-making determine national trajectories.[8] Does the political system, for example, allow interest groups to veto policies that run against their interests? Does it have mechanisms that favour the achievement of consensus-building, and so on? Others[9] place particular emphasis on the theory of path dependence: 'that what happened at an earlier point in time will affect the possible outcomes of a sequence of events occurring at a later point in time'.[10] The idea is there are decisive junctures that condition later events by creating new stakeholders and by setting in train policy feedbacks, related either to popular attitudes or to economic expectations, which then make change to another course more difficult. This framework has been fruitfully applied to China, to explain why retrenchment of government was weaker in urban than rural areas after 1978.[11]

An alternative, recent, approach switches attention from national forces of change to the transnational, attending to ways in which diffusion between countries explains the various shapes of health welfare and services.[12] Lucas[13] and Borowy[14] also described the role of policy diffusion from central and eastern Europe mediated by the Rockefeller Foundation and the League of Nations Health Organization in the development of the health system in China. Using 'interactive diffusion' as a theoretical lens, Hu Aiqun argued that China adopted the Soviet model of social welfare in the early 1950s both to imitate development of a Soviet-style socialist economy and to demonstrate loyalty to the socialist club. Hu argued that the adoption of the Soviet model led to instability of the welfare system, which was significantly changed in the 1960s and 1970s.[15]

Our previous article argued for the importance of a range of factors in generating a path-dependent trajectory of hospital-centrism in China.[16] Highlighting the role of financing, this chapter argues that the impact of industrialisation, historical-institutionalism and diffusion are all helpful in explaining the shaping of China's current hospital-centric health system.

Sources

These arguments are mainly built on four types of sources. First, books on general history of medicine in China such as *The History of Chinese Medicine* (Wong & Wu, 1936) and the works of other historians and social scientists who have studied history on more specific periods or topics provided a chronicle of medicine-related events and their historical contexts. Second, national and local official documentations of history, statistics and compiled policy documents, such as the *China Health Yearbooks* and provincial health gazettes from eastern, central and western China (Shandong, Jiangxi, Guangxi), were selected to complement the national yearbooks. Third, an extensive range of journals and newspapers provided the perspectives of elite Western medicine doctors and other policy actors. Fourth, anthologies, biographies, memoirs and historical studies of important actors (such as Jin Baoshan, who was Director of the National Health Administration during the 1940s) were collected and analysed. Finally, although national archives are inaccessible for post-1949 periods, documents kept in the local archives of Beijing and Pinggu (a suburban district of Beijing and a rural county before 2001) were also searched and used.

In what follows, we work chronologically through the historical evolution of hospitals and primary care providers in China during the three periods from 1835 to 2018, and then wrap up with a discussion of the key historical stages, a brief comparison between China, the United States and the United Kingdom, and the role of financing in the historical process.

The origin of divergence, 1835-1949

In the traditional Chinese medical world, medical services were mainly provided on an ambulatory basis. As we are going to show, the precursory model of hospitals was brought in from Western medicine. As Hu's theory of interactive diffusion suggested, diffused institutional construction needs to respond to local context. During the period from 1835 and 1949, China went through a series of wars, revolutions and fragmentation, including the First Opium War (1839-1842) which opened its closed market, the Boxer Uprising (1899-1901) during which native Chinese rebelled against foreigners, the Xinhai Revolution (1911) which overthrew the imperial system, and the Warlord Era (1916-1928). Hospital-based Western medicine adapted to the historical reality in China upon its introduction and created a set of institutions that consolidated step-by-step the model of hospitals in China over time. In 1928, the Nationalists unified the country and built a central government. The general peace was broken by the Japanese invasion in 1937, dragging the county deeply into the Second World War until 1945, the end of which was immediately followed by a major civil war, then the founding of the People's Republic of China in 1949. For the years between 1928 and 1949, we are also going to show how a model of medical development focusing on primary care was later introduced but was unable to shift the country's health development fundamentally away from hospitals.

The introduction of hospital-based Western medicine

The start of modern medicine in China is usually traced to the Canton Ophthalmic Hospital. This eye hospital was the first Western medicine institution (in Canton, now Guangzhou, Guangdong), and was opened by Peter Parker, a pioneer Christian medical missionary, in 1835. The narrow focus on eye problems was justified as they were among the most common illnesses amongst the Chinese,[17] and effective treatment (i.e. surgery) was not available but could transform patients' lives.[18] The Canton Ophthalmic Hospital became a success and treated more than 900 patients in the first three months.[19] Parker was also active in making known among his foreign sponsors the value of hospitals, and convinced newspaper reporters in England, for example, that his plan for hospitals not only advanced science, but also created good feelings between China and Western powers which facilitated greater engagement with the country.[20]

This was important because the Canton Hospital was built amid grave tension between China and the Western powers on the eve of the First Opium War (1839-1842). Eye surgery was considered an effective way to demonstrate the power of Christianity as well as the technical supremacy of Western civilisation. The hospital, and Parker himself, became an icon for Western engagement with China[21] and prompted the establishment of the Medical Missionary Society in China,[22] and the building of more hospitals in the country after the Opium War.[23] Nevertheless, it was very limited in scale and services. The records of the Canton Hospital during its early years suggested patients were mainly using it for day surgery,[24] and it would also be difficult to establish conclusively the advantage of Western medicine, as it was not until the late nineteenth century when antisepsis and an anesthesia were developed for surgery.[25]

The missionaries over time consolidated a particular model of the hospital in terms of service organisation and financing. They came to the view that hospitals should be the centre of medical missionary work since they enabled lengthy engagement with patients that facilitated religious preaching.[26] The missionaries' guidance also suggests that they valued generalist outpatient care based in hospitals as a way to engage a wider community of potential believers.[27] The consensus around such hospital-centric model incorporating inpatient and general ambulatory care provided the justification for continuous missionary funding input. Furthermore, it allowed hospitals to develop using local sources of funding via substantial outpatient services, revenue from which supported seventy-four per cent of mission hospitals.[28] This was a critical factor, as the rich would try to avoid hospitals. With the expansion of patients' payment, the number of staff in hospitals was several times larger than those in dispensaries by the early 1900s.[29]

As mentioned above, the country was in chaos and fragmentation in the early 1900s. Progress in establishment of health services under the state was limited to either local initiatives or selected sectors (e.g. railways and customs). There was barely any national coordination of medical development by the government, and factions of Western medicine started to emerge because of the difference in training and background between medical missionaries from the West (and their Chinese apprentices) and an increasing number of Chinese medical doctors trained in Japan who were returning to China.[30] The latter had experienced the rapid development of modern medicine in Japan and started to open medical schools teaching Japanese-influenced modern medicine.[38] Their emergence challenged the image of Western medicine and the dominance of medical missionaries, and medical missionaries started to worry about being 'discredited in the eyes of the educated Chinese from a professional standpoint'.[31]

Scientific medicine started to be reinforced within the medical mission. New sources of money emerged, first through an indemnity for missionary hospitals after the Boxer Rebellion, and then via the establishment of the China Medical Board by the Rockefeller Foundation.[32] Benefiting from the newly found resources, and stimulated by rapid medical development in Western countries and China's engagement with Japan, medical professionals became increasingly assertive of professional values and started to demand modernisation of medicine through the building of modern hospitals and high-standard medical schools that could provide proper medical services and conditions for research. Balme wrote a report based on a large-scale survey of mission hospitals, exposing to their funders the poor quality of hospitals, which lacked both proper equipment and qualified staff.[33] The movement towards scientific medicine further consolidated the hospital-centric model by tying it firmly to medical professionalisation.

A report by the China Medical Commission,[34] noted that mission hospitals had most of their non-staff expenditures covered by local sources by 1914. This demonstrated the financial viability of hospitals and was an important factor contributing to the decision to strengthen mission hospitals. The locations of institutions receiving aid from the China Medical Board were thus concentrated mainly in coastal and large cities in alignment with existing missionary medical schools.[35]

In the face of financial difficulty during the Great Depression in the 1930s, Hume, a medical school leader, pushed for the admission of private paying patients.[36] The high cost of hospitals no doubt contributed to the concentration of medical schools and hospitals in large cities. Over time, local resources became critical in hospital financing.[37]

From hospitals to health organisations

A milestone event in extending health services to the mass population occurred with the establishment of the first central health ministry in 1928, when the Nationalist regime unified the country. The founding of the Ministry of Health triggered discussion of 'state medicine'. The idea of state medicine was inspired by the development of social welfare in Western Europe and Soviet Union,[38] but more importantly the emergence of community-based social medicine in eastern Europe.[39] Meanwhile, domestic experimentation with various projects of rural community health care was crucial in forging the agenda of state medicine.[40]

Among the various local experiments, the work of Zhiqian Chen (also known as C.C. Chen) in Ding County, an ordinary poor agricultural county, was the most influential and was directly incorporated in a nation-wide blueprint.[41] In 1932, Chen took charge of Ding County's Department of Rural Health of the Mass Education Movement—an influential rural reconstruction program. Chen conducted a simple economic evaluation of feasible public health interventions that could address the most pressing disease burden of rural populations. He soon realised the limitation of fiscal space—villagers spent only 30 cents (the currency unit was silver dollar—which was a coin made from Mexican silver) on average (based on an earlier survey in Ding

County) on traditional medicine.[42] Chen designed the rural health programme to address the villagers' primary health problems, which were mainly infectious diseases, like smallpox, trachoma, dysentery, tetanus, and typhoid. He found that to address these most pressing needs it was neither feasible nor necessary to rely solely on doctors and nurses.[43]

The model Chen developed was a county-wide multi-tier health organisation approach involving facilities responsible for different levels of care, costing only 9.08 cents annually per capita—less than a third of villagers' annual health expenditure.[44] The health organisations included, from the bottom to the top: village health workers (with 10 days of training and continuous supervision), who provided most of the services for each village (about 1,000 people) and cost only 1.65 cents annually per capita; sub-district health stations (staffed by 'general practitioner[s] for public health'), which provided technical supervision to village health workers and outpatient services for conditions beyond their competence for all sub-district population (about 30,000 people), and cost 3.23 cents; and a county health centre, which provided comprehensive leadership of county-wide health affairs, and supervision and support for village and sub-district health centres, and which was incorporated with a hospital of 30-45 beds, and cost 4.2 cents.[45] There were two key aspects of the cost-effectiveness of the model: on the one hand were the short-term trained local village health workers, who in total cost less than 20% of overall budget. Running each village health station (including remuneration and the cost of drugs, vaccines and other basic supplies) cost only 1% of the budget for a subdistrict health station and only 1/2000 of the budget for a district health centre (including a hospital of 45 beds). The village health stations provided day-to-day management of health of the villagers. On the other hand, the village health workers were reinforced by the sub-district and county health facilities as they formed a multi-tiered referral system. The Ding County Model therefore represented an effort to develop not only a model of primary care providers suitable to rural conditions, but also new roles for hospitals and doctors.

The multi-tier model of Ding County proved impossible to scale up. In 1935, China had only 0.01 Western medical doctors per thousand population as compared to 0.34 per thousand in Yugoslavia, the other classic example of interwar rural social medicine. Furthermore, almost all Western medical doctors 'followed the money' and practiced in large cities.[46] Because of limited resources and government commitment, it was not until the 1940s that the central government started to scale-up state medicine programs and recruit state medical doctors,[47] while efforts to mobilise private practitioners for state medicine were generally unsuccessful.[48] Some county health centres tended to focus on hospital-based curative care for neighboring residents only, rather than supporting the sub-district and village health providers.[49]

After this unsuccessful attempt to shift doctors towards primary care, training of state doctors in the 1940s shifted towards public health. A revised state medicine model, more narrowly focused on prevention than the Ding County experiment, was extended in inland provinces, along with the retreat of the Nationalist regime, during the Second World War.[50] This orientation towards prevention was problematic given the lack of support from hospitals and professional doctors. Some found that such doctors were not competent enough to provide curative services and were therefore unable to win the patient trust needed to deliver public health services.[51]

The period from 1835 to 1949 therefore saw two separate models of health service delivery. Primary care providers and hospitals had their own pattern of service organisation and financing respectively (see Table 7.1). While the model for hospitals was based on medical school-affiliated hospitals transplanted from the West, the primary care model was represented by rural health programmes under the state, influenced by social medicine ideas emerging in central and eastern Europe. The separation of the two models was marked by the failed attempt to scale up a multi-tier design of health services based on the Ding County experiment in the early 1930s. Reorienting the hospitals towards primary care strengthening failed due to the weak financial and regulatory power of the state medicine reformers, particularly given the separate funding bases of the two models.

Table 7.1: Financial sources of hospitals and primary care providers (1928-1949)

	Type of provider	Financial sources	Services
Hospitals	Urban hospitals	Mission Government Private out-of-pocket	Mainly curative
Primary care providers	Urban private practitioner	Urban private out-of-pocket	Mainly curative
	State medicine sub-district health stations	Government	Mainly preventive, curative
	Village health workers	Rural community	Mainly preventive

Source: authors

Establishing socialist medicine, 1949-1978

From 1949 to 1978, the Communist government took strong control of health services, recognising them as a major social project in its effort to build a socialist industrialising state. As industrialisation developed in urban areas, the rural economy was developed based on collective agriculture. A two-tier economic and social welfare system was formed, where urbanites enjoyed substantially more benefits than their rural counterparts.[52] This structural reality affected the evolution of hospitals and primary care providers from 1949 to 1978. The early split in trajectories developed further. The 1950s was marked with a diffusion of Soviet model of health services, which further changed the balance of care and tilted it towards urban hospitals. The efforts to shift services towards primary care took place most evidently in rural areas and became embedded in the rural socio-economy.

Adapting the Soviet model of health services

In the years after 1949, leaders of the newly founded People's Republic of China decided to organise its urban health sector following the Soviet model of health service organisation, as part of a wider effort to adopt Soviet experiences of national development.[53] Two major urban insurance schemes, namely the Labour Insurance Scheme (LIS, covering formal industrial employees) and the Government Insurance Scheme (GIS, covering governmental and para-governmental employees and students) were established in 1951 and 1952 respectively, drawing on Soviet model.[54] Due to scant financial resources, only enterprises with 100 or more employees were covered by LIS.[55] While the LIS was funded by premiums collected from factories, the GIS was budgeted along with other government health expenditure.[56] The Nationalist government hospitals and mission hospitals started to be nationalised, enhanced, and the distribution of health care service became more evenly spread.[57] The Soviet model of shorter medical education with earlier specialisation was also adopted, while medical schools were reformed, created and redistributed across the country.[58] 19,770 students were enrolled at medical schools in 1951, dwarfing the accumulated number of medical graduates over the previous seven decades.[59] Thus the development of urban hospital financing (urban insurance schemes and out-of-pocket payments of urban patients) extended the pre-1949 medical school-based model of hospitals by adopting the Soviet system.

Hospital care soon became unaffordable for the new socialist state, as deficits in the insurance schemes emerged shortly after their establishment. GIS and LIS spending quickly surpassed the growth rate of the overall economy.[60] Growing hospital deficits were reported across the country.[61] For example, insurance scheme-affiliated institutions of the Shandong Provincial Government had increasing deficits in the GIS from 18% of fund budget in 1954, 33% in 1955 and 42% in 1956.[100] With weak administrative capacity, the excessive use of services and medicines covered by the insurance funds was widely reported.[62]

The Ministry of Health (MOH) and local health agencies responded with attempts to bring down the cost. First, a Soviet-style referral system called 'sectional health care' (*diduan yiliao*) was introduced to facilitate the coordination of care across hospitals and primary care facilities. In essence, this was another attempt to build a multi-tier referral system, this time where the primary care facilities functioned as the gatekeepers and higher-level facilities provided care to referred patients. However, the municipal health agency in Beijing reported that patients did not trust primary care facilities and patients still preferred to go to 'large hospitals'.[63] Second, hospitals were required to expand less costly services, including outpatient care and prevention.[64] The MOH required hospitals to function as centres for preventive services, although this was a political requirement not followed by corresponding financial reward.[65]

Third, the government also reinforced subsidy for hospitals with two other initiatives. Salaries of hospital staff were no longer to be recovered from service revenue but fully budgeted and covered by the government.[66] Also, the difference between wholesale and retail prices of pharmaceuticals was to be used to subsidise hospitals so that hospitals could 'purchase [pharmaceuticals] at the wholesale prices and sell at retail prices to patients'.[67] The principle of service price reduction was 'less reduction for outpatient care, more reduction for inpatient care; less reduction for ordinary medical services, more reduction for surgeries, in order to reflect the spirit of less reduction for minor conditions and more reduction for serious conditions'.[68] Therefore, outpatient user fees and pharmaceutical sales became further institutionalised as important ways to subsidise hospital services.

None of these efforts were enough to reduce the expenditure on LIS and GIS. Over time, the risk pool for LIS collapsed and the scheme became solely based on individual enterprises.[69] The 'wasteful' use of fund-covered services and medicines was considered a constant problem facing GIS—the fund was eventually separated from the overall health budget in 1980.[70] Industrial health service providers continuously expanded in numbers of facilities, except during the recession after the Great Leap Forward.[71] As a result, it was never really likely that coverage under the two schemes would be extended to cover rural health services.

Rural health services and cooperative medicine

In rural areas, a different kind of state medical planning was introduced. This included the restoration and construction of county health centres and sub-district health stations, training village health workers as well as the retraining of midwives to provide modern midwifery.[72] The government allowed the continuation of private practice and group practices (essentially fee-for-service).[73] In return, health committees and associations of private practitioners were organised locally below the level of the county to ensure they carried out epidemic prevention and control, as well as maternal and child health work, under the supervision of local health centres and stations.[74] The government made it clear that the main concern for rural areas was prevention.[75] This focus was considered reasonable as prevention was more challenging in rural areas due to such problems as illiteracy, superstition and poor transportation.[76]

The issue of providing curative care to the rural population soon emerged. During the late 1950s, agricultural collectivisation started to develop rapidly in rural China, providing both political justification and a collective financial base to develop medical risk pooling. The first Cooperative Medical Scheme (CMS) was established in 1955.[77] Then a nationwide campaign was organised to promote CMS during the Great Leap Forward movement, but the scheme then collapsed following the fall of the movement.[78] Group practices (mainly union clinics) were made public and became the commune health centres, and later *township* health centres as communes were transformed into townships. The MOH, under tight fiscal constraints, was generally cautious in extending financial coverage for curative care in rural areas and repeatedly argued that grassroots health facilities should be allowed to charge user fees and not hastily become public providers of free care (see Table 7.2). Although the MOH tended to emphasise the role of county hospitals (the medical arm of the county health centres that became independent), the government eventually provided a 60% subsidy for the commune/township health centres. Meanwhile, the county health bureaux assumed responsibility for their administration.[79]

The lack of health care benefits for the rural population became unacceptable to Chairman Mao, who launched a reprimand condemning the MOH for neglecting rural health care and called for a shift of focus to the countryside on 26 June 1965. Two years after the start of the

Cultural Revolution in 1966, Mao openly endorsed the CMS and 'barefoot doctors'. This quickly led to scaling up of the CMS nationwide and its continuance until the late 1970s.[80] The CMS was mainly based on funds extracted from collective agriculture.[81] The barefoot doctors were peasants who completed a very brief training in medicine and undertook primary health care services at the village level, while still participating in collective agricultural work and earning work-points for their medical activities as members of the community.[82] Urban doctors were sent to county hospitals and commune health centres in large numbers, providing training for rural barefoot doctors. For example, in the two years of 1969 and 1970, 30% of total medical staff in Beijing were sent to settle in rural or remote areas.[83]

Just like the LIS and GIS, the CMS faced constant challenges of deficit, despite the fact that government lowered the prices of hospital services.[84] Sources from the Pinggu County Archive show that in 1972, 51.03% of cooperative medical stations were in deficit.[85] In 1974, the central government directly provided subsidy for the CMS.[86] However, still more than a third of cooperative medical stations were almost bankrupt by 1978.[87] With scant and unstable revenue from agricultural yield, a political campaign was launched to reconstruct the value of local resources—such as replacing Western pharmaceuticals by Chinese herbal medicine locally produced by agricultural collectives. For instance, the CMS in Pinggu County built 67 native pharmacies during the early 1970s,[88] and patients were encouraged to use these herbal medicines.[89]

The CMS thus relied on collective funds to subsidise pharmaceuticals and referral to hospital, collective work to subsidise production of local herbal medicines, and collective agriculture (where health service was just one component of labour) to finance the barefoot doctors. Although the rural health services were supported by staff from the urban areas, these doctors' participation was not institutionalised financially or organisationally. Therefore, although the rural health services in the late 1960s and 1970s had a multi-tier structure, the linkages between the hospitals and primary care facilities were very weak and highly dependent on the social circumstances of the Cultural Revolution.

As the MOH had weak control of local health facilities, staff with little training were also recruited into the township health centres.[90] Medical education was also reformed so that medical schools stopped producing university-degree graduates and instead produced graduates with only three-years training, who were later found to be poorly skilled.[91] These policies were not only to prove unsustainable but also created serious challenges for the future. Rather than consolidating primary care as a professional equivalent to hospital care, they generated a cohort of primary care doctors below the standard needed to lead primary care.

Overall, a fragmented financing structure emerged in China's health system, which both shaped and was shaped by the service-delivering facilities from 1949 to 1978. The Soviet model provided the initial framework of health financing and delivery. However, the model was too expensive for China, and therefore did not expand widely to cover peasants. When the government tried to reform the system and shift focus to rural areas, the highly constrained fiscal space of rural areas led to the development of rural primary care that was weakly institutionalised, underfinanced, and still not far advanced from its original private orientation.

Table 7.2: Policy statements on ownership of and financial responsibility for primary care facilities

Year	Policy
1957	'union clinics [group practices of mainly private practitioners] emerged from the people… are health welfare institutions with socialist nature, the state should not take them over'[a]
1959	'for the medical expenditures of the people… it is best to mainly rely on individual payment, with appropriate subsidy from the state and communes'[b]
1960	'collective health and medical schemes are considered preferable'[c]
1962	'the main form of rural grassroots health organizations should be doctor-owned group practices for a very long period of time'[d]
1965	'doctors' group practices are the most numerous and the most problematic, and should gradually move towards commune/brigade ownership'[e]
1974	'the policy of 'commune sponsorship with public aid' applies for collectively-sponsored commune health centres'[f]

Sources:
a. Ministry of Health, 'Directive on Strengthening Leadership of Grassroot Health Organisations', in *Collection of Rural Health Policy Documents (1951-2000)*, ed. by Keling Liu Changming Li, Zhaoyang Zhang, Chunlei Nie, Wei Fu, Hongming Zhu, Bin Wang (Department Grassroot Health and Maternal and Child Health, Ministry of Health, 1957).
b. ———, 'Opinions on Several Issues Regarding Health Work in People's Communes (*Guanyu Renmin Gongshe Weisheng Gongzuo Jige Wenti De Yijian*) (in Chinese)', (1959).
c. ———, 'Report on the National Rural Health Field Conference in Qishan, Shanxi (*Guanyu Quanguo Nongcun Weisheng Gongzuo Shanxi Qishan Xianchagn Huiyi Qingkuang De Baogao*) (in Chinese)', (1960).
d. ———, 'Opinions on Improving Several Issues Related to Hospital Work *(Guanyu Gaijin Yiyuan Gongzuo Ruogan Wenti De Yijian)* (in Chinese)', (1962).
e. ———, 'Report on Putting the Stress of Health Work in Rural Areas (*Guanyu Ba Weisheng Gongzuo Zhongdian Fangdao Nongcun De Baogao*) (in Chinese)', (1965).
f. Ministry of Health, *op. cit.* (note 86).

Reform and re-reform (1978-2018)

The period between 1978 and 2018 saw rapid and stable growth of the Chinese economy. China's industrialisation reached a new height and it became one of the world's leading manufacturing powers. This period saw a U-turn in public share (represented by government finance and social input—predominantly social health insurance in Figure 1) in overall health financing, which declined continuously for two decades before rising in the latter one and a half decades. Introduction of market-based financing mechanisms brought direct competition between hospitals and primary care providers and exposed the weakness of the latter. The links that connected the hospitals and primary care providers were essentially broken. After 1978, pharmaceuticals and technologies became critical vehicles for hospitals' revenue generation. Resources that became increasingly available due to the rise of the Chinese economy were absorbed primarily by hospitals, while the primary care sector struggled to secure a model of financing that allowed its sustainable development.

Figure 7.1: Composition of sources of total health expenditures in China from 1978 to 2016

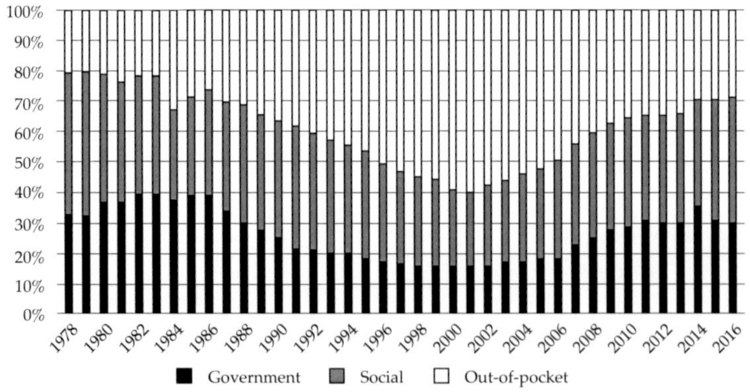

Data source: National Health and Family Planning Commission, *China Health and Family Planning Statistical Yearbook 2017* (Beijing: Beijing Union Medical University Press, 2017).

Seeking revenue from market

The post-1978 reform brought challenges and new opportunities for financing both hospitals and primary care facilities. The reform started with decollectivisation of agricultural production which led to the collapse of the collective agricultural system that financed the work of barefoot doctors. The CMS also collapsed, largely because of a backlash against the ideology to which the CMS was tied during the Cultural Revolution.[92] Contemporary studies by researchers also highlighted the importance of local political leadership in determining CMS success.[93] At the central level, the worry about heavy financial burden of peasants and the tense relationship between local government (township and village) and peasants made the government reluctant to push harder for the resurrection of CMS in the 1990s.[94] Local governments were responsible for public expenditure on local health facilities, but they were predominantly concerned with economic growth and cut down on their health spending.[95] Urban enterprise-based welfare also encountered difficulties: as a result of the reform of state-owned enterprises during the post-1978 economic reform, businesses had to bear the consequences of economic losses. The state-owned enterprises were allowed to be privatised or closed, leading to the laying-off of many workers, who thus lost their entitlement to health benefits.[96]

The government was committed to the maintenance and modernisation of health facilities,[97] which required additional resources. As government financial input and insurance fund payments continued to drop as a percentage of overall health expenditures (see Figure 7.1), a main concern of policymakers was the financial deficits of health facilities, particularly urban hospitals which faced expanding demand.[98] The two issues were seen as related, as the lack of incentive due to poor cost recovery was considered a contributor to low service provision.

The central government and the MOH used two main approaches to seek additional revenue for health facilities from the market.

First, the price schedule was reformed. Low charges for hospital services were the result of the 1960 policy of government subsidy to physician salaries, which was believed not to have been well implemented: prices were reduced for both patients and insurance funds but not with a parallel increase in salary subsidy.[99] With declining government share in health financing, this price system had to be changed. However, the simultaneous reduction of social health insurance meant that increasing the price of medical services systematically would impose a heavy financial burden on those not covered by public health insurance.[100]

The government adopted new policies to allow hospitals to increasingly rely on private payment and revenue generated through expensive services. In 1981, the State Council approved a dual fee schedule, allowing hospitals to charge GIS and LIS patients at cost of services while keeping the prices for other urban residents and the rural population unchanged.[101] In 1985, the government again allowed price increases for new equipment, new medical procedures, and newly built, renovated and expanded facilities, and reemphasised the need for separate fee schedules for insured and uninsured patients, while again avoiding general adjustment of prices.[102] In 1996, the government further pushed for increased cross-subsidy from high technology services through higher charges which were then redistributed among the hospitals.[103] Although the policy document admitted the problem of encouraging excessive sales of expensive pharmaceuticals, the policy makers did not remove pharmaceutical mark-up, knowing that there would be no alternative revenue source.

Second, the State Council also implemented a management responsibility system for hospital economic operations.[104] In effect, hospitals were supposed to cross-subsidise among their own services:

non-basic services could be provided with a profit margin, while basic services were to be provided below cost.[105] The result was a rapid growth of pharmaceutical expenditures, which was particularly fast in inpatient services (see Figure 7.2). Official documents noted that hospitals borrowed heavily in order to purchase expensive equipment,[106] and regional quotas were exceeded.[107] Hospital debt increased much faster than assets and revenues.[108]

Figure 7.2: Pharmaceutical expenditures on outpatient and inpatient care

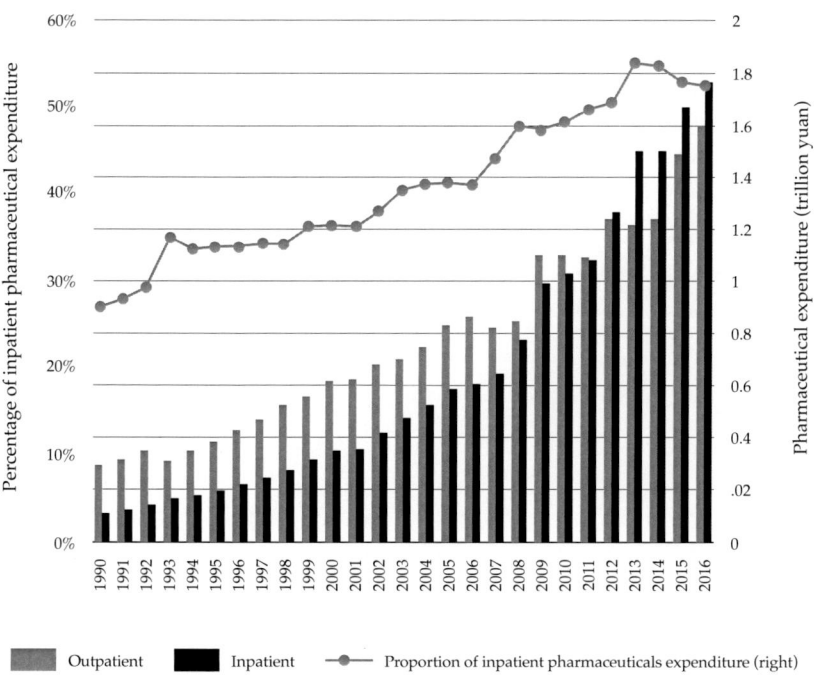

Sources: authors.

The commercialisation of the hospitals was accompanied by the decline of the publicly-funded primary care sector, which had never been strongly embedded. Barefoot doctors had to rely on user fees paid by the peasants. The number of barefoot doctors started to decline, as their main source of revenue shifted to drug sales,[109] and many left the ranks. About half of the 1.2 million that remained passed a certification process and became village doctors, while the other half became village health workers.[110] In 1985, the term barefoot doctors ceased to be used.[111] The village doctors also tended then to neglect preventive services.[112]

The township health centres struggled to retain doctors, as their weak revenue basis was exposed when central financial subsidy and dispatch of urban doctors dwindled. The withdrawal of 'sent-down' hospital doctors became a common phenomenon. Local reports suggested that the conscripted doctors almost completely left township health centres: for example in the early 1980s, 166 technical 'backbones' (most of whom had been sent down from urban hospitals) left the health services of Pinggu, Beijing, destroying its technical capacity.[113] In a township health centre in Liaoning, only one out of 11 specialised secondary school graduates sent to work there from 1962 remained working there in 1982, while more than two thirds of its staff were temporary.[114] Some of the local health administrators said the rural health professionals were being 'eradicated'.[115] Those who exited tended to be the more qualified professionals. Financial concerns were critical drivers of the exodus of doctors, along with other non-financial issues such as lack of career prospects.[116]

The inheritance of unqualified, even semi-illiterate workers from the Cultural Revolution period up until the early 1980s, and the retirement of doctors trained before 1949, meant that many township health centres were far from ready to compete in the market. The only exception were those who had been able to develop specialties.[117] In other words, there was no sustainable financial model or fiscal space for primary care. Fee for service payment further undermined the development of general practice, as the focus of primary care providers shifted towards curative care with neglect of prevention.

Towards universal health coverage

Around the turn of the century, China's poor health risk-pooling was exposed by the WHO *World Health Report 2000*, prompting a more assertive approach by the state towards population coverage and access.[118] In 1998, the LIS had been restructured as an urban insurance scheme for employees. In 2002 and 2005, two other extensive social health insurance schemes were established and started expanding. The three schemes and GIS eventually covered the whole population. The government started to invest in public health services on both demand- and supply-sides. In 2009 (a few years after the outbreak of Severe Acute Respiratory Syndrome (SARS) in 2002) the government launched a reform to provide basic universal health coverage. The increase in government and social (i.e. premium collected from employers and employees) financing was conspicuous (see Figure 1).

What did this mean for hospitals, primary care, and the balance between them? The three social health insurance schemes expanded in population coverage and fundraising, leading to a decline in out-of-pocket payments as a share of total health expenditure from 60% in 2001 to 37.5% in 2009 and further to 28.8% in 2016 (see Figure 1).[119] Besides the expansion of insurance, the reform in the early 2000s covered four other main areas: essential medicines, essential public health services, service delivery (focusing on primary care), and public hospitals.[120] All of the reforms included a financing element. The essential medicines policy required zero-price mark-up in pharmaceutical dispensing and replaced it with a set fee for each consultation, which removed the strong incentive to generate income through prescribing excessively. The essential public health services programme had a new benefit package and designated capitation-based funding. The service delivery reform replaced previous revenue-based salaries with a rigid but generally low salary, which seem ineffective in incentivising medical services. While these reform policies were launched in primary care facilities shortly after the 2009 health system reform, it took more than a decade to remove the drug mark-up in public hospitals.[121] The payment for hospital services was still primarily fee-for-service and reform for hospitals and hospital-based physicians were also patchy and mainly local. Hospitals' incentive to pursue revenue generation remained unchanged. This drove rapid accumulation of resources in hospitals, reinforcing the financial disadvantage of primary care.

With the essential public health services programme, primary care facilities started to receive a capitation-based budget for providing a package of essential public health services, separate from the social health insurance schemes which covered inpatient and outpatient services. There was some evidence that low salary and rigid policy targets related to non-clinical service procedures were demotivating for providers, nor did the reform resonate with patient's preferences for care.[122] The visits to primary care providers as a proportion of overall visits continued to decline. From 2004 to 2016, the number of visits to primary care facilities increased from 2.58 billion to 4.37 billion, a 69 % increase, while visits to hospitals increased from 1.3 billion to 3.27 billion or by 152%.[123]

As a result of the asymmetric timing of reforms, from 2009 hospitals grew ever more dominant in health financing (see Figure 7.3). By contrast, township health centres as well as primary care facilities overall experienced much slower increase in revenue. One particular phenomenon was the rise of county hospitals. County hospitals received support from the government because they were recognised as the local centre to provide technical leadership for the rural multi-tiered health services. Indeed, the years after 2009 saw the rapid catching up of county hospitals with urban hospitals (see Figure 7.3). Among all hospitals, those with more than 800 beds grew the fastest, from 180 in 2002 to 1,602 in 2016 or by 8.9 times, compared to 1.6 times growth of all other hospitals; specialist hospitals also grew faster than general hospitals.[124] Larger hospitals also provided an increasingly large share of overall hospital beds—the proportion of total beds in hospitals with more than 500 beds increased from 41% in 2002 to 52% in 2016 (see Figure 7.4). The particularly rapid development of large hospitals and specialised hospitals suggests that the current model rewards increased specialisation of clinical services.

Figure 7.3: Health expenditures by types of facility (adjusted to 1990 price level)

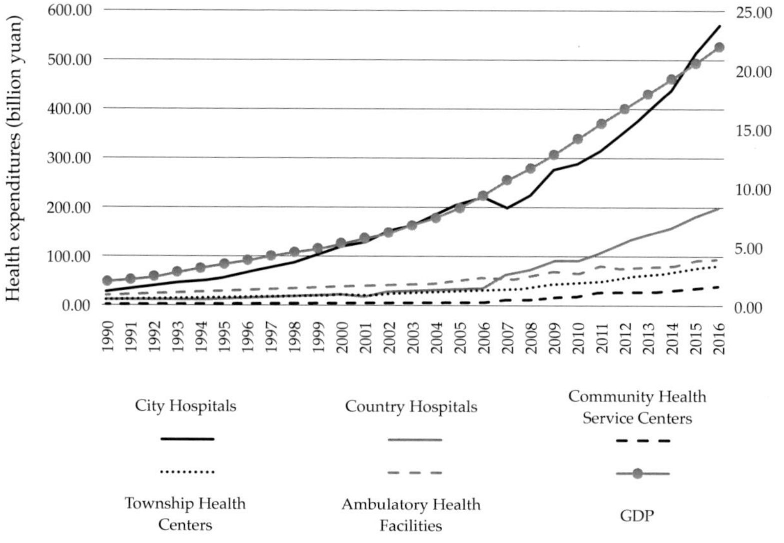

Source: Authors' calculation from data from the China National Health Development Research Center, *op. cit.* (note 119).

Figure 7.4a: Number hospitals classified by size (number of beds) (2002 and 2016)

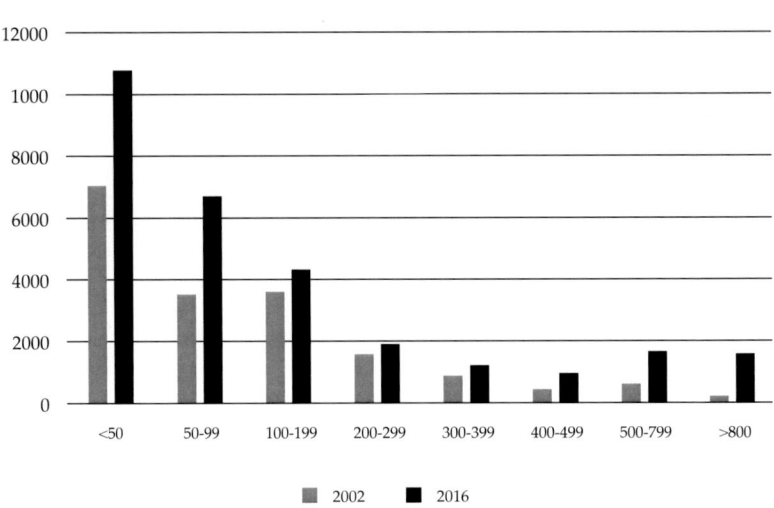

Sources: Authors' calculation from data from:
———, *op. cit. (note 160)*.
National Health and Family Planning Commission, *China Health and Family Planning Statistical Yearbook 2017* (Beijing: Beijing Union Medical University Press, 2017).

Figure 7.4b: Estimated proportion of beds in hospitals classified by size (number of beds) (2002 and 2016)

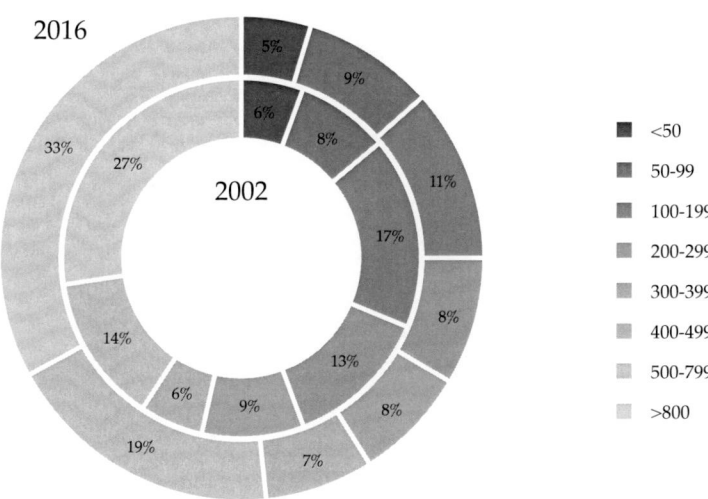

Sources: Authors' calculation from data from:
———, *op. cit. (note 160)*.
National Health and Family Planning Commission, *China Health and Family Planning Statistical Yearbook 2017* (Beijing: Beijing Union Medical University Press, 2017).

Note: As the yearbooks cited here only reported average number of beds in each size category (e.g. hospitals with 100-199 beds), we estimated proportion of beds in hospitals classified by size. Number of beds of hospitals with fewer than 800 beds were calculated using the number of hospitals multiplied by the mid-point of the range of number of beds in each category shown in the figure. Number of beds of hospitals with more than 800 beds were calculated using the total number of hospital beds minus the total of beds of hospitals with fewer than 800 beds.

Discussion

We have surveyed the historical evolution of financing for hospitals and primary care facilities in China from 1835 to 1949. Here we summarise the key historical stages and discuss the role of financing in the historical evolution of the balance between hospital and primary care.

Summary of key historical stages

Fiscal space in China before 1949 was extremely limited, inhibiting the growth of a public hospital system. The period 1835-1928 saw the rise of mission hospitals (incorporating substantial ambulatory care) as the dominant form of Western medicine supported by external funding sources and local revenue largely via outpatient care. From 1928 to 1949, a social medicine movement plotted a diverging trajectory of low-cost primary care. While the original plan was to reposition hospitals and doctors so as to strengthen primary health services provided mainly by lay health workers, the limited fiscal and regulatory capacity led to separation of hospitals from primary care facilities focused primarily on public health services. While the model of the medical-school-affiliated hospital was diffused directly from the West, the primary care model after 1928 was also heavily influenced by international practice, despite substantial local adaptation.

In the 1950s, hospitals were reinforced through the development of urban medical insurance schemes based on Soviet practice as well as fees from private paying urbanites. Specialist-oriented educational reform combined with an expansion of hospital-based ambulatory care further undermined the potential for primary care financing to develop based on general practice. The model was too expensive for the young and mainly agricultural country, leaving the majority population—the peasants—without coverage. The pre-1949 model of focusing on public health services within primary health care was initially adopted during the early 1950s. Then it became unacceptable that the rural population could not enjoy health risk pooling like urban dwellers. Primary care was implemented nation-wide with central subsidy and mobilisation of professionals from hospitals in support, through training, sustained clinical guidance and even staffing. However, it remained constrained as local health providers still relied on meagre and unstable agricultural revenues during the late 1960s and the 1970s.

After 1978, market-based financing reforms introduced direct competition between hospitals and primary care providers, which exposed the weakness of the latter. Pharmaceuticals and technologies became critical vehicles for hospitals' revenue generation. Primary care suffered from chronic funding shortages. The post-2002 expansion of social health insurance schemes for urban and rural residents channeled funds disproportionately to hospitals. The much longer delay in reforming financing in hospitals as compared to primary care also suggested a stronger resistance to change.

Health financing history and hospital centrism

The effects of structural factors, diffusion and path dependent processes all seemed important in generating the historical institutions that underpin China's contemporary hospital-centrism, which not only provided limited value of health services despite rapidly increasing cost, but also proved difficult to change. The theories can complement each other and provide a comprehensive explanation for the evolution of the balance of hospitals and primary care.

Structural factors played an obvious role. For example, the overall lack of financial resources and the gap between urban and rural socio-economic development up to 1978 affected the shaping of primary care which aimed at extending health care coverage to the vast rural population. Separated, differentiated and tiered financing contributed to the divergent institutionalisation of hospitals and primary care facilities over the long term.

Policy diffusion was also important. The rise of Western medicine hospitals in China involved the adoption of an American model of academic hospitals by philanthropists and a Soviet model supported by public health insurance. Apart from such bilateral diffusion, the later primary care movements were also affected by the transnational diffusion from the social medicine practiced in central and eastern Europe mediated by international organisations such as the Rockefeller Foundation and the League of Nations Health Organisation.

What we have demonstrated is that historical structural factors (such as the limited fiscal space due to lack of economic development) and diffused policy models (such as the establishment of Flexner-inspired elitist medical universities in China) were embedded in the historical institutions that affected later periods, even when the structural factors were modified and the diffused model became outdated. As in China, primary care strengthening has been a late comer in many low- and middle-income countries, which face the similar challenge of hospital-centrism based on models diffused from developed countries. The 1930s and 1960s marked two important periods when the two-model system of diverging hospitals and primary care facilities was formed. The relative success in the latter period relied heavily on the ability of government to mobilise professionals from hospitals to support primary care through training, sustained clinical guidance and referral. This was however unsustainable and undermined by the reform after 1978, as hospitals needed to generate revenue in competition with primary care providers. Although reforms could relatively quickly increase public financial input, their effects might also be circumscribed by the long-term shaping effects of earlier financing policies. Thus, historical institutionalism is helpful to explain why it was so hard to create a primary-care-centric health system in all three periods (1835-1949, 1949-1978 and 1978-2018).

This chapter has highlighted the role of historical fiscal space in shaping the development of the service model of health facilities. This is supported by previous historical work in wealthy countries. In the United States, the emergence of privately-paying patients contributed to the specialisation of medical services and the rise of hospitals over primary care facilities.[125] In the United Kingdom, the early empanelment of doctors to provide general medical care, based on the National Health Insurance Act of 1911, provided a stronger institutional basis for primary care to consolidate financially and professionally.[126] Furthermore, we also hinted at the difficulty of transforming the complex financing system underpinning hospitals and primary care providers in China. The way health facilities were funded profoundly affected the positioning of service delivery. Revenue generation policies under tight fiscal constraints could create resistance to redirection of resources. This is illustrated by the long delay in adjusting price schedules and removing pharmaceutical mark-up in China in recent years.

Conclusion

A health system focusing on hospital care is associated with high cost as well as suboptimal health outcomes. As China experiences rapid population ageing and a sharp increase in a non-communicable disease burden, the importance of a primary-care-centred health system to provide continuous, coordinated and cost-effective services has become an imperative and has been well recognised by both the national government and key international agencies. Understanding the historical path that has led to the current uneven balance of care is important in framing our understanding of contemporary challenges facing primary care strengthening and developing solutions.

We have analysed the historical coevolution of primary care facilities and hospitals in China from 1835 to 2018, focusing on the role of financing in shaping the historical trajectories of hospital-centrism despite multiple waves of primary care strengthening. While hospitals consolidated their revenue-generation and service dominance over time, the late development of financing policies and fiscal space for primary care constrained its institutionalisation. As resources became increasingly abundant, they were increasingly allocated to hospitals while primary care continued to be poorly supported. For contemporary policies, a key implication is that these historically conditioned methods of financing health care institutions need to be understood, so that the resourcing of hospitals and primary care providers can become better aligned in order to drive them to work together towards primary care strengthening.

1. JX was funded by the China Scholarship Council 'National Graduate Students Programme for Constructing Advanced Universities' (201206010317) and Peking University Health Science Center grant (BMU2017YB006). The funding bodies did not participate in the design of the study and collection, analysis, and interpretation of data nor in writing the manuscript. Materials were mainly drawn from Jin Xu's PhD thesis work at London School of Hygiene & Tropical Medicine, when he was supervised by Prof. Anne Mills and advised by Prof. Martin Gorsky.

2. Kenneth W. Newell, Health by the People (Geneva: World Health Organization, 1975).

3. J. Xu, and A. Mills, 'Challenges for Gatekeeping: A Qualitative Systems Analysis of a Pilot in Rural China', Int. J. Equity Health, 16 (2017), 106; Jin Xu, Martin Gorsky, and Anne Mills, 'Historical Roots of Hospital Centrism in China (1835–1949): A Path Dependence Analysis', Social Science & Medicine, 226 (2019), 56-62.

4. Jin Xu, op. cit. (note 3), 56-62.

5. Theda Skocpol, Peter Evans, and Dietrich Rueschemeyer (eds), Bringing the State Back In: Strategies of Analysis in Current Research (Cambridge: Cambridge University Press, 1999).

6. Jacob S. Hacker, 'The Historical Logic of National Health Insurance: Structure and Sequence in the Development of British, Canadian, and Us Medical Policy', Studies in American Political Development, 12 (1998), 57-130.

7. Peter A. Hall, and Rosemary CR Taylor, 'Political Science and the Three New Institutionalisms', Political Studies, 44 (1996), 936-57; Theda Skocpol, and Edwin Amenta, 'States and Social Policies', Annual Review of Sociology (1986), 131-57; Theda Skocpol, Peter Evans, and Dietrich Rueschemeyer, op. cit. (note 5).

8. Ellen M. Immergut, 'Institutions, Veto Points, and Policy Results: A Comparative Analysis of Health Care', Journal of Public Policy, 10 (1990), 391-416; Sven Steinmo, and Jon Watts, 'It's the Institutions, Stupid! Why Comprehensive National Health Insurance Always Fails in America', Journal of Health Politics, Policy and Law, 20 (1995), 329-72.

9. Jacob S. Hacker, op. cit. (note 6), 57-130; Paul Pierson, 'Increasing Returns, Path Dependence, and the Study of Politics', American Political Science Review (2000), 251-67.

10. William H Sewell, 'Three Temporalities: Toward an Eventful Sociology', in T.J. McDonald (ed), The Historic Turn in the Human Sciences (Ann Arbor: University of Michigan Press, 1996), 245-80.

11. Jane Duckett, The Chinese State's Retreat from Health: Policy and the Politics of Retrenchment (London: Routledge, 2012).

12. Mary Brown Bullock, An American Transplant: The Rockefeller Foundation and Peking Union Medical College (Berkeley: Univ. of California Press, 1980).

13. AnElissa Lucas, Chinese Medical Modernization: Comparative Policy Continuities, 1930s-1980s (New York: Praeger, 1982).

14. Iris Borowy, 'Thinking Big--League of Nation's Efforts Towards a Reformed National Health System in China', in Iris Borowy (ed), Uneasy Encounters: The Politics of Medicine and Health in China 1900-1937, (Fraunfurt am Main, Germany: Peter Lang, 2009), 205-28.

15. Aiqun Hu, 'China, Social Insurance and the Welfare State: A Global Historical Perspective', World History Connected, 9, 1 (2012).

16. Jin Xu, op. cit. (note 3), 56-62.

17. Later in the influential rural health survey in Ding County, acute conjunctivitis and trachoma were found to be the most prevalent conditions among villagers and included as priority conditions for treatment in the rural health programs Zhiqian Chen, 'Dingxian Shehui Gaizao Shiye Zhong Zhi Nongcun Weisheng Shiyan (Fubiao), 'Rural Health Experiment in the Social Reconstruction in Ding County (with Attached Tables)', Weisheng yuekan (Health Monthly), 4 (1934).

18. Jonathan D. Spence, 'Peter Parker: Bodies or Souls', in Jonathan Spence, To Change China: Western Advisers in China, 1620-1960 (New York: Penguin Group, 1969), 34-56.

19. Jonathan D. Spence, op. cit. (note 18), 34-56.

20. Peter Parker, Statements Respecting Hospitals in China--Preceded by a Letter to John Abercrombie, M.D., V.P.R.S.E, (Glasgow: Medical Missionary of the American Board of Foreign Missions in China, 1842); Spence, op. cit. (note 18), 34-56.

21. Spence, op. cit. (note 18), 34-56.

22. T. R. Colledge, Peter Parker, and E. C. Bridgman, 'Suggestions for the Formation of a Medical Missionary Society Offered to the Consideration of All Christian Nations, More Especially to the Kindred Nations of England and the United States of America', in The Medical Missionary Society in China: Address with Minutes of Proceedings, Etc., Etc. (Canton, 1838: 1835).

23. Peter Parker, op. cit. (note 20).

24. Qizi Liang, 'The Birth of Modern Chinese Hospitals (Jindai Zhongguo Yiyuan De Dansheng) (in Chinese)', in Yiping Zhu (ed), Jiankang Yu Shehui: Huaren Weishegn Xinshi (Health and Society: New History of Chinese Health) (Taiwan: Linking Publishing, 2013), 41-68.

25. Harold Ellis, A History of Surgery (Cambridge: Cambridge University Press, 2002).

26. Conference Committee, China Centenary Missionary Conference Records--Report of the Great Conference Hold at Shanghai, April 5th to May 8th, 1907 (New York: American Tract Society, 1907).

27. Harold Balme, China and Modern Medicine (London: United Council for Missionary Education, 1921).

28. Michelle Campbell Renshaw, Accommodating the Chinese: The American Hospital in China, 1880-1920 (Adelaide: University of Adelaide, 2003), 148-72.

29. Conference Committee, op. cit. (note 26).

30. ———, 'Si, Jiuzhongguo De Xiyi Paibie Yu Weisheng Shiye De Yanbian (Part Four, Factions of Western Medicine and Evolution of Health Services in Old China)', in Jin Baoshan Wenji (a Collection of Jin Baoshan's Work), ed. by Yanjie Mo, Yude Chen, Rui Li and Jun Zhong (Beijing: Beiyi Gongwei 'Xiyanghong' Bianjizu ('Red Setting Sun' Editorial Group, School of Public Health, Beijing Medical University, 2007), 92-99.

31. Harold Balme, op. cit. (note 27); Paul U Unschuld, Medicine in China: A History of Ideas. Comparative Studies of Health Systems and Medical Care (Berkeley: University of California Press, 1985).

32. Tietao Deng, and Zhifan Cheng, Jindai Juan (Modern Times Volume) (in Chinese). In Weikang Fu, Jingwei Li and Zhaogeng Lin (eds), Zhongguo Yixue Tongshi (a General History of Chinese Medicine) (in Chinese) (Beijing: People's Medical Publishing House, 2000); K. Chimin Wong, and Lien-teh Wu, History of Chinese Medicine--Being a Chronicle of Medical Happenings in China from Ancient Times to the Present Period (Shanghai, China: National Quarantine Service, 1936).

33. Harold Balme, op. cit. (note 27).

34. China Medical Commission of the Rockefeller Foundation, Medicine in China (The University of Chicago Press, Chicago, Illinois, U.S.A., 1914), 113.

35. Rockefeller Foundation, The Rockefeller Foundation Annual Report 1922, (New York: Rockefeller Foundation, 1922).

36. Edward H. Hume, 'The Place of Mission Hospitals and Medical Schools in the National Health Programme of China', Chinese Medical Journal, 49 (1935), 946-50.

37. Szeming Sze, China's Health Problems (Washington, D.C.: Chinese Medical Association, 1943), 60.

38. Mary Brown Bullock, op. cit. (note 12).

39. Iris Borowy, op. cit. (note 14), 205-28; Lien-teh Wu, 'Altruism in the Medical Profession', The National Medical Journal of China, 47 (1931), 268-82.

40. Sean Hsiang-lin Lei, Neither Donkey nor Horse: Medicine in the Struggle over China's Modernity (University of Chicago Press, 2014).

41. Baoshan Jin, 'Gongyi Zhidu (State Medicine)', Xingzheng yanjiu (Administrative Studies), 1 (1936), 129-33.

42. C. C. Ch'en, 'Scientific Medicine as Applied in Ting Hsien: Third Annual Report of the Rural Public Health Experiment in China', The Milbank Memorial Fund Quarterly Bulletin, 11 (1933), 97-129.

43. Zhiqian Chen, 'Dingxian Shehui Gaizao Shiye Zhong Zhi Nongcun Weisheng Shiyan (Fubiao) '(Rural Health Experiment in the Social Reconstruction in Ding County (with Attached Tables)', Weisheng yuekan (Health Monthly), 4 (1934), 9-18.

44. C. C. Chen, 'The Rural Public Health Experiment in Ting Hsien, China', The Milbank Memorial Fund Quarterly, 14 (1936), 66-80.

45. C. C. Chen, op. cit. (note 44), , 66-80; ———, 'Some Problems of Medical Organ-

isation in Rural China', Chinese Medical Journal, 1937 (1937), 803-14; ———, 'State Medicine and Medical Education', Chinese Medical Journal, 49 (1935), 951-54.

46. ———, op. cit. (note 44), 951-54; Hsi-Ju Chu, and Daniel G. Lai, 'Survey Distribution of Modern-Trained Physicians in China', Chinese Medical Journal, 49 (1935), 542-52.

47. ———, 'Sanshi Nian Lai Zhongguo Gonggong Weishegn Zhi Huigui Yu Qianzhan (Public Health in China over the Past 30 Years and Its Prospects)', National Medical Journal of China, 32 (1946).

48. Li Qian, 'Wuguo Tuixing Gongyi Zhidu Zhi Kunnan Yu Cuowu (Daixu) (Difficulties and Mistakes in Implementing State Medicine in China (to Be Continued))', Shehui weisheng (Social Hygiene), 2 (1947), 1-4; Szeming Sze, op. cit. (note 37), 60.

49. R. K. S. Lim, and C. C. Chen, 'State Medicine', Chinese Medical Journal, 51 (1937), 781-96; Andrija Stampar, 'Health and Social Conditions in China', Quarterly Bulletin of the Health Organization of the League of Nations, 5 (1936), 1090-126.

50. Xi Gao, 'Between the State and the Private Sphere: The Chinese State Medicine Movement, 1930-1949', in by Liping Bu, Darwin H. Stapleton and Ka-Che Yip (eds), Science, Public Health and the State in Modern Asia (London: Routledge, 2012).

51. Li Qian, op. cit. (note 48), 1-4.

52. Yifu Lin, 'Ganchao Zhanlue He Chuantong Jingji Tizhi (Catching-up Strategy and Traditional Economic System)', in Zhongguo Jingji Zhuanti (on Chinese Economy) (Beijing: Peking University Press, 2008), 307.

53. Aiqun Hu, op. cit. (note 15).

54. Government Administration Council of the Central People's Government, 'Directive on Implementing Publicly Funded Medical Care and Prevention for Nationwide State Employees in All Levels of People's Government, Parties, Groups and Affiliated Public Institutions', (1952); ———, 'Implementation Measures of Publicly Funded Medical Care and Prevention for State Employees ', (1952); ———, Zhonghua Renmin Gongheguo Laodong Baoxian Tiaoli (People's Republic of China's Regulations on Labour Insurance) (in Chinese)', (1951).

55. Aiqun Hu, op. cit. (note 15).

56. Xinzhong Qian, Zhongguo Weisheng Shiye Fazhan Yu Juece (The Development and the Strategy-Making of China's Health Work) (in Chinese) (Beijing: Zhongguo yiyao keji chubanshe (China Medicine Technology Press, 1992).

57. ———, 'Guanyu Zhengdun Quanguo Yiyuan De Zhishi (Directives on Rectifying Hospitals Nationwide)', (1950).

58. ———, 'Zhongyang Renmin Zhengfu Weishengbu Gongbu Quanguo Weisheng Dahui Guanyu Yiyao Jiaoyu Deng Sixiang Jueding (Central People's Government Issued Four Decisions of the National Health Congress Regarding Medicines, Education, Etc)', Traditional Chinese Medicine Journal (1951), 1-5; ———, 'Zhongguo Weisheng Guanli De Lishi Jingyan (Historical Experience in Health Management in China) (in

Chinese)', Chinese Social Medicine (1988); Xuewen Zhang, Xinzhongguo De Weishegnshiye (Health Affairs of the New China) (in Chinese) (Beijing: Shenghuo·Dushu·Xinzhi Sanlian Shudian (Life Reading New Knowledge Three-United Bookstore), 1953.

59. People's Daily, 'Quanguo Tuixing Xinyixue Jiaoyu Zhidu Huoude Chengji, Jinnian Yixuexiao Jiuxuezhe Chaoguo Yiwang Liushijiu Nian Suo Xunlian De Yisheng Zongshu (Nationwide Implementation of New Medical Education System Achieve Good Results, Students in Medical Schools across Nation Has Exceeded Total Number of Doctor Trained over Past 69 Years) (in Chinese)', People's Daily, 3 November 1951.

60. Hongqing Liu, ' Gongfei Laobao Yiliao—Jianxing Jianyuan De Jiyi (Government Insurance Medical Scheme and Labour Insurance Medical Scheme--Increasingly Distant Memories) (in Chinese)', Chinese Social Security (Zhongguo Shehui Baozhang), 11 (2009), 121.

61. Wenjun Wu, ' Xinzhongguo Chuqi Gongfei Yiliao Zhidu Jianshe Yanjiu--Jiyu Fan Langfei De Shijiao (The Study of Construction of the Public Health System in the Early New China-Based on the Perspective of Anti-Waste) (in Chinese)', Jingji Jishu Yu Guanli Yanjiu (Technological Economy and Management Studies) (2014), 86-90.

62. Wenyong Cao, 'Zhizhi Gongfeiyiliao Zhong De Yanzhong Langfei (Stopping the Serious Waste in Publicly Funded Medical Care) (in Chinese)', Renmin Ribao (People's Daily), 10 September 1955; Yun Huang, 'Dangqian Gongfei Yiliao Jingfei Guanli Zhong De Wenti He Gaijin Yijian (Issues and Opinions on Improvement of the Current Fund Management of Publicly Funded Medical Care (in Chinese)', Caizheng (Finance) (1957), 15-17; Ruiqing Liu, 'Gongfei Yiliao Zenyang Cong Chaozhi Bianwei Youyu (How to Turn Deficit of Publicly Funded Medical Care into Surplus) (in Chinese)', Caizheng (Finance)(1957), 32; Yi Yin, 'Kefu Gongfei Yiliao Zhong De Langfei Xianxiang (Overcoming the Phenomena of Waste in Publicly Funded Medical Care) (in Chinese)', Renmin Ribao (People's Daily), 8 January 1955.

63. Beijing Municipal Public Health Bureau, 'Guanyu 'Fenji Fengong Yiliao' Gongzuo Zhong Ruogan Wenti De Shuoming (Explanations Regarding Several Issues in the Work Related to 'Stratified and Divided Medical Services')' (1956).

64. ———, Zonghe Yiyuan Gongzuo Zhidu, Zonghe Yiyuan Gongzuo Renyuan Zhize (Work Regulations for Comprehensive Hospitals, Staff Responsibility for Comprehensive Hospitals) (Beijing: People Health Publishing House, 1958).

65. Yi Yin, op. cit. (note 62).

66. Biao He, Autobiography of He Biao (He Biao Huiyilu) (in Chinese) (Beijing: Chinese People's Liberation Army Publishing House (Jiefangjun Chubanshe), 2001); Ministry of Health, and Ministry of Finance, 'Joint Circular Regarding That Expenditures on Hospital Staff Wages Becomes Full-Budgeted by the State (Guanyu Yiyuan Gongzuo Renyuan De Gongzi Quanbu You Guojia Yusuan Kaizhi De Lianhe Tongzhi) (in Chinese)', (1960).

67. Ministry of Health, and Ministry of Finance, op. cit. (note 66) (1960).

68. Ministry of Health, and Ministry of Finance, op. cit. (note 66) (1960).

69. Aiqun Hu, op. cit. (note 15).

70. Xinzhong Qian, op. cit. (note 56).

71. ———, 'Health Statistics Information in China 1949-1988', (1989).

72. ———, 'Nongcun Weisheng Jiceng Zuzhi Gongzuo Juti Shishi Banfa (Cao'an) (Detailed Implementation Plan of Work on Rural Health Organization (Draft))', in Keling Liu Changming Li, Zhaoyang Zhang, Chunlei Nie, Wei Fu, Hongming Zhu (eds), Collection of Rural Health Policy Documents (1951-2000), Bin Wang (Department Grassroot Health and Maternal and Child Health, Ministry of Health, 1951), 241-51; ———, 'Directives on Medical Administration Work This Year', Shandong Zhengbao (Shandong Policy Paper) (1950), 81; Xinhua Agency, 'Quan'guo Nongcun Weisheng Jiceng Zuzhi Xunsu Kuozhan (Rapid Expansion of Rural Health Organisations across the Country) (in Chinese)', Renmin Ribao (People's Daily), 1951.

73. ———, op. cit. (note 56), 241-51.

74. Nianqun Yang, Remaking 'Patient': Spatial Politics under the Conflicts between Chinese and Western Medicine, 1832-1985 (China Renmin University Press, 2006).

75. ———, op. cit. (note 56), 241-51; ———, op. cit. (note 71), 81.

76. Qin Zhang, ' Guanyu Nongcun Weisheng Jianshe Wenti--Ji Zhongyang Weishengbu Nongcun Weisheng Zuotanhui (On Constructing Rural Health Services--Notes of Rural Health Forum of Central Ministry of Health) (in Chinese)', Renmin Ribao (People's Daily) 1950.

77. ———, 'Guanyu Woguo Nongcun Hezuo Yiliao Baojian Zhidu De Huiguxing Yanjiu (a Retrospective Study of the Rural Cooperative Medical Scheme of China) (in Chinese)', in On Cooperative Medicine (Beijing: China Rural Medicine Publishing House, 1993).

78. Yaowen Yi, 'Jishanxian De Nongcun Weisheng Baojian Wang (Rural Health Care Network in Jishan County) (in Chinese)', Renmin Ribao (People's Daily) 1958.

79. D.M. Lampton, The Politics of Medicine in China: The Policy Process, 1949-1977 (Boulder: Westview Press, 1977).

80. ———, op. cit. (note 80).

81. ———, 'Macheng Xian Hezuo Yiliao Zanxing Guanli Banfa (Shixing Caoan) (Temporary Regulations for the Coperative Medical Scheme in Macheng County (Trial Draft))', in Qinli Nongcun Weishegn Liushi Nian (Experiencing 60 Years of Rural Health Services) (in Chinese) (Beijing: Peking Union Medical College Press, 1966), 300-03.

82. Dan Hu, Weiming Zhu, Yaqun Fu, Minmin Zhang, Yang Zhao, Kara Hanson, Melisa Martinez-Alvarez, and Xiaoyun Liu, 'Development of Village Doctors in China: Financial Compensation and Health System Support', International Journal for Equity in

Health, 16 (2017), 9.

83. Beijing Municipal Health Bureau, 'Benju Guanyu Jiaqiang Nongcun Weisheng Gongzuo, Nongcun Yiliaodui Jiti Renyuan Zhuanwei Guojia Zhigong Deng Gongzuoe De Qingshi, Baogao (The Bureau's Proposal and Report on Reinforcing Rural Health Work and Converting Collective Members of Rural Medical Team into State Employees) (in Chinese)' (1973).

84. Ministry of Health, and Ministry of Finance, op. cit. (note 66).

85. Pinggu Health Bureau, 'Health Statistics Report 1973' (1973).

86. Ministry of Health, '1973 Nian Quanguo Jiaoyu Weishegn He Xingzheng Zuotanhui Fujian San Guanyu Weisheng Shiye Jihua Caiwu Gongzuo Zhong Ruogan Wenti De Yijian (Zhaiyao) (1973 National Administrative Group Discussion on Education and Health, Third Attachment--Opinions Regarding Issues in Health Affairs Planning and Financial Work) (in Chinese)' (1974).

87. ———, 'Health Statistics Report 1979' (1979).

88. ———, Pinggu Health Gazette (1986).

89. Party Branch of Heidouyu Brigade at Huangsongyu Commune, 'Jianchi Sixiang Zhengdun, Jianshe Geminghua Weishengyuan (Holding on to Thought Correction, Building Revolutionized a Health Centre) (in Chinese)' (1977).

90. Zikuan Zhang, 'Cong Yifeng Xiang Weishengyuan Zhang De Laixin Tan Nongcun Weishengyuan De Gaige Wenti (Discussing the Reform of Rural Health Centers in Relation to a Letter Sent from the Director of a Rural Township Health Center)', in Lun Hezuoyiliao (on Cooperative Medicine) (Beijing: China Rural Medicine Publishing House, 1984).

91. Zhuofu Luo, and Jingyao Sun, Beijing Yike Daxue De Bashinian (the Eight Decades of Beijing Medical University) (Beijing: Peking University Medical Press, 1992).

92. ———, 'Zai Hezuoyiliao Wenti Shang Yinggai Chengqing Sixiang Tongyi Renshi (Understanding About Cooperative Medicine Should Be Clarified and Consolidated)', in Lun Hezuoyiliao (on Cooperative Medicine) (Beijing: China Rural Medicine Publishing House, 1987).

93. Gerald Bloom, and Shenglan Tang, Health Care Transition in Urban China (Gower Publishing, Ltd., 2004).

94. Shaoguang Wang, 'Adapting by Learning: The Evolution of China's Rural Health Care Financing', Modern China, 35 (2009), 370-404.

95. Jane Duckett, op. cit. (note 11).

96. Jane Duckett, op. cit. (note 11).

97. ———, op. cit. (note 93).

98. State Council, 'Guowuyuan Pizhuan Weishengbu Guanyu Weisheng Gongzuo Gaige Ruogan Zhengce Wenti Baogao De Tongzhi (Circular on Approving and Forwarding Ministry of Health's Report on Several Policy Issues Related to Health Work Reform) (in Chinese)' (1985)

99. ———, 'Guowuyuan Pizhuan Weisheng Bu Jiejue Yiyuan Peiben Wenti De Baogao (State Council's Circular on Approving and Ministry of Health's Report Regarding Solving the Problem of Economic Loss of Hospitals) (in Chinese)' (1981).

100. Winnie Yip, and Karen Eggleston, 'Addressing Government and Market Failures with Payment Incentives: Hospital Reimbursement Reform in Hainan, China', Social Science & Medicine, 58 (2004), 267-77.

101. National Planning Commission, Ministry of Health, and Ministry of Finance, 'Guanyu Jiaqiang He Gaijin Yiliao Fuwu Shoufei Guanli De Tongzhi (Circulation on Strengthening and Improving Management of Medical Service Charges)' (1996).

102. ———, 'Weishengbu Guanyu Kaizhan Weisheng Gaige Zhong Xuyao Huaqing De Jitiao Zhengce Jiexian (On Several Policy Boundaries That Need Clarification in Implementing Health Reform) (in Chinese)' (1985).

103. ———, op. cit. (note 101).

104. State Council, op. cit. (note 99).

105. X. Liu, Y. Liu, and N. Chen, 'The Chinese Experience of Hospital Price Regulation', Health Policy Plan, 15 (2000), 157-63.

106. National Planning Commission, Ministry of Health, and Ministry of Finance, op. cit. (note 101).

107. Shixue Li, 'The Problems of Hospital Reimbursement and Related Suggestions', (Jinan: 1997).

108. National Health and Family Planning Commission, Ministry of Finance, State Commission Office for Public Sector Reform, National Development and Reform Commission, Ministry of human Resources and Social Security, State Administration of Traditional Chinese Medicine, and State Council Office of Health Reform, 'Guanyu Quanmian Tuikai Gongli Yiyuan Zonghe Gaige Gongzuo De Tongzhi (Announcement on Rolling-out Comprehensive Reform of Public Hospitals in All Aspects)', (2017).

109. Gerald Bloom, 'Primary Health Care Meets the Market in China and Vietnam', Health Policy, 44 (1998), 233-52.

110. Duckett, op. cit. (note 11).

111. ———, China Health Yearbook 1988 (Beijing: People's Medical Publishing House, 1988).

112. X. Liu, and W. C. Hsiao, 'The Cost Escalation of Social Health Insurance Plans in China: Its Implication for Public Policy', Soc Sci Med, 41 (1995), 1095-101.

113. ———, op. cit. (note 86).

114. Xingzhu Liu, Lingzhong Xu, and Shuhong Wang, 'Reforming China's 50 000 Township Hospitals—Effectiveness, Challenges and Opportunities', Health Policy, 38 (1996), 13-29.

115. ———, 'Guanyu Jiaqiang Nongcun Weisheng Duiwu De Guanli He Jishu Peixun Wenti—Dongbei Sansheng Nongcun Yiliao Weisheng Jianshe Diaocha Zhi San (on Strengthening Management of Rural Health Workforce and Professional Training—Rural

Health Construction Investigation in the Three Northeast Provinces, No. 3', Nongcun Weisheng Shiye Guanli Yanjiu (Rural Health Service Management Research) 2 (1982).

116. Ibid.

117. Zikuan Zhang, 'Cong Yifeng Xiang Weishengyuan Zhang De Laixin Tan Nongcun Weishengyuan De Gaige Wenti (Discussing the Reform of Rural Health Centers in Relation to a Letter Sent from the Director of a Rural Township Health Center)', in Lun Hezuoyiliao (On Cooperative Medicine) (Beijing: China Rural Medicine Publishing House, 1984).

118. World Health Organization, The World Health Report 2000: Health Systems: Improving Performance (WHO, 2000).

119. China National Health Development Research Center, 'China National Health Accounts Report 2017', (2017).

120. Central Committee of Communist Party of China, and State Council, 'Guanyu Shenhua Yiyao Weisheng Tizhi Gaige De Yijian (Opinions on Deepening Health System Reform)'2009) [Accessed 6 February 2013].

121. ———, 'Guowuyuan Guanyu Yinfa Yiyao Weishegn Tizhi Gaige Jinqi Zhongdian Shishifangan (2009-2011nian) De Tongzhi (the State Council's Circular Regarding the Implementation Plan for Key Points of Health System Reform in the near Future (2009-2011))' (2009); National Health and Family Planning Commission, op. cit. (note 108).

122. J. Xu, and A. Mills, op. cit. (note 3), 106.

123. National Health and Family Planning Commission, China Health and Family Planning Statistical Yearbook 2017 (Beijing: Beijing Union Medical University Press, 2017).

124. ———, China Health Statistical Yearbook 2003 (Beijing: Peking Union Medical College Publishing House, 2003); National Health and Family Planning Commission, op. cit. (note 108).

125. Charles E. Rosenberg, 'The Private Patient Revolution', in The Care of Strangers: The Rise of America's Hospital System (New York: Basic Books, 1987).

126. Frank Honigsbaum, The Division in British Medicine: A History of the Separation of General Practice from Hospital Care, 1911-1968 (London: London School of Economics and Political Science, 1979).

Biographical Notes on Contributors

Barry Doyle is Professor of Health History at the University of Huddersfield. He is an expert on the history of European hospitals, healthcare and the city in the nineteenth and twentieth centuries. His work has received funding from the Wellcome Trust, the Arts and Humanities Research Council and various community and academic organisations including the Heritage Lottery Fund. He has published extensively on the history of hospitals and healthcare in Britain, France and Central Europe, including a monograph, *The Politics of Hospital Provision in Early Twentieth Century Britain*. In addition to a number of chapters in edited collections he has been published in a variety of journals including *Social History of Medicine, Medical History, Historical Research, Revue d'histoire de la protection sociale* and *Urban History*. Between 2015 and 2019 he was a co-editor of *Cultural and Social History*. He is currently editing a special issue of *European Review of History* with Hannah-Louise Clark entitled *Imperial and Post-Imperial Healthcare before Welfare States*.

Martin Gorsky is Professor of History in the Centre for History in Public Health at the London School of Hygiene and Tropical Medicine. His early research examined the roles of philanthropy and mutualism in the British hospital and social security system prior the National Health Service (NHS). He has since researched and published widely on different aspects of public health and health systems, including: the financing and geography of British hospitals before and after the coming of the NHS; patterns of morbidity during the English mortality transition and the response of the friendly societies; the public health poster in Poland; administration and management in the NHS; and public health in English, and particularly London's, local government. He currently holds a Wellcome Trust Investigator Award, which is examining the intellectual and policy history of 'health systems', viewed from the perspective of international organisations and through country case studies.

Frank Grombir, BA, MA, PGCert, AFHEA specialises in the study of migration, diasporas and national identity in 20th century Britain and Central and Eastern Europe. He worked as a research assistant on the European Healthcare before Welfare States project at the University of Huddersfield between 2016 and 2017 and is currently completing a Ph.D. in History at the University of Hull supervised by Dr Nicholas Evans and Dr Catherine Baker. His public history engagement in the Kirklees area has included numerous history talks and walks, journal editorship, community partnership projects and heritage events.

Melissa Hibbard, BA, MA, PhD, is a historian of health with a focus on early twentieth century Poland. She completed her doctorate at the University of Illinois, Chicago on Children of the Polish Republic: Child Health, Welfare, and the Shaping of Modern Poland, 1914-1938 in 2020. Melissa currently works as a History teacher in Montana, USA.

Beatrix Hoffman is Professor in the Department of History at Northern Illinois University. She has published *Health Care for Some: Rights and Rationing in the United States since 1930*, The University of Chicago Press, 2012; Co-editor with Nancy Tomes, Rachel Grob, and Mark Schlesinger, *Patients as Policy Actors*, Rutgers University Press, 2011; and *The Wages of Sickness: The Politics of Health Insurance in Progressive America*, The University of North Carolina Press, 2001. Her work has received support from the Robert Wood Johnson Foundation, the National Endowment for the Humanities, and the American Council of Learned Societies. She is currently working on a history of immigrant rights to health care in the U.S.

Axel C. Hüntelmann is Postdoctoral Research Fellow at the Institute for the History of Medicine at the Charité Medical School in Berlin, where he is currently part of a project on brain research at Kaiser-Wilhelm-Institutes between 1939 and 1945. Previously, he has worked and published on the German Imperial Health Office (PhD 2007) and other European public health institutions between 1850 and 1950; scientific infrastructures; the history of laboratory animals; the production, clinical testing, marketing, and regulation of pharmaceuticals in Germany and France; and he has written a biography on the immunologist Paul Ehrlich (2011). He trained in accounting as well as history and is currently finishing a book on accounting and bookkeeping in medicine (1730–1930). Recently, he has edited (together with Oliver Falk) a volume on *Accounting for Health. Calculation, paperwork and medicine, 1500-2000* (Manchester University Press, 2021).

Anne Mills is Professor of Health Economics and Policy at The London School of Hygiene & Tropical Medicine (LSHTM) and has been Deputy Director & Provost since 2012. She studied history and economics at the University of Oxford, and completed her PhD at LSHTM on the economics of malaria. She is a worldwide authority on health economics and health systems research, with a particular focus on how to create efficient and equitable health systems in low- and middle-income countries. She has held the position of President of the International Health Economics Association, and has been board member of Health Systems Global. She received a CBE for services to medicine in 2006, and is a Fellow of the UK Academy of Medical Sciences, US National Academy of Medicine, and the Royal Society. In 2015 she was awarded a DCMG in recognition of her services to international health.

Ana Nemi is Associate Professor of Contemporary History at the Federal University of São Paulo. Her research studies aspects of charity and philanthropy in the history of public health and the organization of hospitals. Among her recent publications are: *Caravans from Escola Paulista de Medicina to Araguaia and Xingu: Medical narratives of expeditions from the 1960s* (Editora da Unifesp, 2020) and *Between public and private - Hospital São Paulo and Paulista School of Medicine (1933 to 1988)* (Editora Hucitec, 2020).

Balázs Szélinger, PhD (b. 1969). Born in a family of medical doctors and pharmacists, he studied History and Mediterranean Studies at the University of Szeged, Hungary (MA and PhD). Formerly an Assistant Professor of History at Mekelle University (Tigray, Ethiopia), a freelancer journalist, and many more, he is recently the Economic and Trade Attaché at the Embassy of Hungary in Addis Ababa, Ethiopia. His research interests include the relations between the Horn of Africa and Central Europe, the modern history of Hungary, and the anthropology of hard rock and heavy metal music.

Margarita Vilar-Rodríguez (University of A Coruña) and **Jerònia Pons-Pons** (University of Seville). Both are professors of economic history and have worked together over the last decade on topics related to public and private health care and hospital coverage in Spain in a comparative perspective with other countries. As a result of this joint work, they published the book *El seguro de salud privado y público en España. Su análisis en perspectiva histórica* (Zaragoza: Prensas Universitarias de Zaragoza, 2014), which received the 2015 Vicens Vives Award for the best Economic and Social History book published in Spain and Latin America; and the book *Un siglo de hospitales entre lo público y lo privado (1886-1986) [Financiación, gestión y construcción del sistema hospitalario español]* (Madrid: Marcial Pons, 2018). Within this line of research, they also published chapters in collective works such as, for example, 'Economic Growth and Demand for Health Coverage in Spain: The Role of Friendly Societies (1870-1942)', in Harris, Bernard (ed.), *Mutual insurance, sickness and old age in Europe and North America since 1850* (London, Pickering & Chatto Publishers, 2012). They have published extensively on these topics, including articles in *International Review of Social History* (2011); *Social History of Medicine* (2012); *Labor History* (2012 and 2020); *Business History* (2019); *The Economic History Review* (2019), *The European Journal of Health Economics* (2019), among others. Together, they organised the International Workshop 'Construction, funding and management of the public and private hospital systems of developed countries' (Seville, 2018) that gave rise to this book. They currently lead the research project entitled *The historical keys of hospital development in Spain and its international comparison during the twentieth century* (Ref. RTI2018-094676-B-I00), that is financed by the Spanish Government's Ministry of Economy and Competitiveness and ERDF funds.

Jin Xu is currently lecturer at Peking University, China, Center for Health Development Studies in Beijing, China. He recently earned his PhD at the London School of Hygiene & Tropical Medicine, with previous undergraduate and graduate training in medical English, economics and sociology at Peking University. He is mainly interested in the transition of health systems and evaluation from multi-disciplinary perspectives. He used historical analysis to understand the roots of weak primary care in the context of China, and demonstrated the added value of a historical perspective to quantitative and qualitative analysis of contemporary primary care. His research interests also include people-centred integrated care, telemedicine as a health system intervention, comparative studies of health systems and health equity. He is leading several research projects related to health system reform in China, with grants from funders including the National Natural

Science Foundation of China. He has published about 20 papers in top international and Chinese journals on medicine and health policy, such as *BMJ, Lancet, Social Science and Medicine, Health Policy and Planning*. Jin Xu is also an editorial advisor for the journal *Health Policy and Planning*, a board member of the Emerging Voices for Global Health, and a fellow of the Equity Initiative (2018-2019).